Ketogenic Bible: The Complete Ketogenic Diet for Beginners - The Only Keto Guide You Will Ever Need

Christine Bailey

Published by Imaginarium Press Publishing, 2019.

While every precaution has been taken in the preparation of this book, the publisher assumes no responsibility for errors or omissions, or for damages resulting from the use of the information contained herein.

KETOGENIC BIBLE: THE COMPLETE KETOGENIC DIET FOR BEGINNERS - THE ONLY KETO GUIDE YOU WILL EVER NEED

First edition. February 27, 2019.

ISBN: 978-1798513897

Written by Christine Bailey.

Also by Christine Bailey

Intermittent Fasting For Women: Powerful Strategies To Burn Fat & Lose Weight Rapidly, Control Hunger, Slow The Aging Process, & Live A Healthy Life As You Keep Your Hormones In Balance

Ketogenic Snacks: Delicious and Ready-to-Go Desserts, Sweets, & Treats to Maintain Ketosis & Keep You Satisfied

Ketogenic Bible: The Complete Ketogenic Diet for Beginners - The Only Keto Guide You Will Ever Need

Keto Meal Prep: Comprehensive Step-by-Step Beginner Guide to Prep, Pack, & Store Low -Carb, High -Fat Ketogenic Recipes for Rapid Weight Loss

Introduction – What is Keto?

THIS BOOK CONTAINS information intended to help readers be better-informed consumers of health care. It is presented as general advice on health care. This book is not intended to be a substitute for the medical advice of a licensed physician. The reader should consult with his/her doctor in any matters relating to his/her health.

The simplest explanation is that a ketogenic diet is a high-fat, low-carbohydrate, and medium-protein diet. The diet became popular as a way to treat refractory epilepsy in children. It makes the body burn fat instead of carbs for energy.

The carbohydrates most people consume are converted to glucose, which the body transports around and which is important for fueling the brain's functioning. However, if the body doesn't have many carbohydrates, the liver will convert fats in the body into fatty acids and ketone bodies. The ketones will then make their way to the brain to replace the glucose. This increased level of ketones helps reduce the frequency of epileptic seizures.

Nearly half the children placed on this diet experienced a reduction in seizures. The effects continued even once they returned to a normal diet.

A classic keto diet contains about a four-to-one ratio by weight of combined carbohydrates and protein to fats. This is done by eliminating high-carbohydrate foods like sugar, grains, pasta, bread, starchy vegetables, and fruits. In addition, the consumption of butter, cream, and high-fat nuts is increased.

Most fats found in food are LCTs or long-chain triglycerides. However, MCTs (short for medium-chain triglycerides) are more ketogenic. Many people who follow a ketogenic diet will use a lot of coconut oil because it's high in MCTs, or they will purchase MCT oil and add it to their coffee in the morning.

Everybody's needs and bodies are different. However, the macro makeup of a keto diet is normally 60 to 75 percent of calories coming from fat, 15 to 30 percent from protein, and five to 10 percent from carbs.

After a few days on the diet, the body will enter what is known as ketosis, which we will go into later. This is when the body starts using stored and consumed fats for energy.

While this diet was originally used to treat epilepsy, people started noticing how useful it was for losing weight. When you consume carbs, the body will hold onto fluids so that it can store carbs for energy. When you don't consume as many carbs, you will lose all the stored water.

The main reason why people start a diet is to get rid of fat stores, and this diet literally targets those stores.

While the diet may seem hard to stick to because it cuts out many foods, there are several creative ways to ensure that you don't miss out on tasty meals. If you stick with it, you'll notice your waistline shrinking in no time.

Speaking of foods, lots of products are aimed toward keto fans. FATBAR is one of them. The company makes snack bars that have 200 calories, four net grams of carbs, and 16 grams of fat.

Those who love coffee and are used to having vanilla lattes every morning can turn to bulletproof coffee. This is regular coffee with butter and MCT oil mixed in.

Let's dive into how to get started.

Starting a Keto Diet

THE KETOGENIC DIET is often shortened to just "keto." The word "keto" comes from the fact that the diet makes your body create small fuel molecules known as ketones. Once glucose is in short supply, your body uses ketones as an alternative fuel source.

When you eat a few carbs, ketones are produced. This is also true when protein intake is kept to a moderate amount. Excess protein can also be turned into sugar.

The liver creates ketones from your fat stores. Ketones will then be used as fuel throughout the different areas of your body as well as by the brain. The brain tends to use a lot of energy every day, but it's not able to run off fat. It is able to get energy only from glucose or ketones.

When you follow a ketogenic diet, your entire body will change its fuel supply so that it runs almost entirely on fats. Your insulin levels will drop, and your fat burning will increase. The body will find it easier to access your fat stores to burn them. This is perfect when you are trying to drop weight; however, there are plenty of other, less obvious, benefits, like a steady energy supply, less hunger, and mental alertness.

How Low Is the Amount of Carbs?

The only way this diet works is if you eat very few carbs. The fewer carbs you consume, the more effective the diet will be at promoting weight loss. A ketogenic diet is an extremely strict low-carb diet. You will consume only 20 grams or less of net carbs every day.

Once you reach your weight loss goals, you can start increasing your carb intake. Do this slowly so you don't gain back the weight.

The Basics

While this may be a great diet, there is a right way and a wrong way to follow it. Make sure you start the right way so that you get better and faster results.

In theory, a keto diet is fairly simple: low carbs, high fat. However, that doesn't really let you know what you can and can't eat. I'll provide a full list of foods you can and can't eat, but right now here's a basic list of what you can eat:

- Heavy fats such as olive oil, bacon fat, tallow, lard, ghee, butter, and coconut oil
- Meats (including organ meats)
- Eggs
- Seafood and fish
- Non-starchy vegetables (you will definitely want leafy greens)
- Some berries, like blueberries, strawberries, and raspberries

This means a typical day could look like:

- Breakfast: Bacon and eggs
- Lunch: Chicken salad with a cup of bone broth
- Dinner: Steak with a side of veggies and a ketogenic dessert

Some people like to have snacks in between their meals. Good ideas include nuts, cheese sticks, broth, celery sticks, and meat sticks. Watch all the snacks, though, as they do add to your total macro count.

The keto diet is also very easily personalized. You can experiment to see what works best for you. Some people find that they need more fat in their diets, while others are able to eat a few more carbs. Some people try intermittent fasting.

Most people who practice intermittent fasting will skip breakfast and have their first meal at one. This ups your ketosis power.

Macros

I've already mentioned macros. You're probably wondering what they are. When used in the contest of the keto diet, "macros" is short for "macronutrients."

Macros are the parts of the food that provide you with energy and fuel. They are fats, carbohydrates, and protein. These are where all your dietary calories come from. If you want to succeed at following a keto diet, it's important that you completely grasp the concept of macros. They must be in the right balance for you to stay in ketosis.

Carbohydrates are the only macro that you don't have to consume in order to survive. There are essential amino acids and fatty acids that are the building blocks of proteins and fats, but there aren't any essential carbohydrates.

Carbs are made up of two things: starches and sugars. Fiber is viewed as a carb, but with a keto diet, it isn't counted in the total carb intake. The reason why is that the body doesn't really digest fiber; therefore, it doesn't have much of an effect on your blood sugar.

This means when you are looking at a nutrition label, you should first look at total carbs, and then at fiber. Subtract the amount of fiber from the total carb amount. This will give you the net carb count.

Total carbs – fiber = net carbs

This means net carbs include only the starches and sugars in the carbohydrates. When you are figuring your macros for a meal, you will use only these net carbs. You do not have to use total carbs.

To succeed, you will want to find foods that are naturally low in carbohydrates and those that aren't. Not all of them are obvious. Of course, potatoes are high in carbs, but did you realize that bananas are high in carbs as well?

People who are starting out on a keto diet should aim to consume around 20 net grams of carbs each day.

Protein is important to the body because it helps preserve lean muscle mass, makes enzymes and hormones, and promotes immune function, tissue repair, and growth. Protein plays a significant role in biological processes. Proteins are known as the building blocks for a healthy body.

When consumed, proteins are broken into amino acids. Nine of those cannot be produced by the body. This is why these essential amino acids must come from foods. These nine are: valine, tryptophan, threonine, phenylalanine, methionine, lysine, leucine, isoleucine, and histidine. When there is a deficiency in protein or any of these amino acids, the result can be kwashiorkor, malnutrition, or several other health problems.

When following a keto diet, you must consume enough protein to preserve your lean body mass. How much you consume will depend on your current amount of lean body mass. Here's a guideline:

- 0.7 to 0.8 grams of protein per pound of muscle to preserve your muscle mass.
- 0.8 to 1.2 grams of protein per pound of muscle to increase your muscle mass.

You never want to lose body mass – only gain or preserve it. Many people focus only on losing weight. However, often, losing weight means losing muscle as well as fat. The goal must be to lose fat and save your muscle. This is important for a person to maintain good metabolism.

Don't go too crazy when you consume protein while on keto. Too much could stress your kidneys and also affect ketosis. Try to keep your macros in the ranges suggested above.

Let's look at an example:

Let's assume you weigh 160 pounds and have 30 percent body fat. This means you have around 48 pounds of body fat. You can subtract your body fat from your total weight. This will give you your lean body mass. In this instance, it would be 112 pounds.

To figure out how much protein you should consume, take the lean body mass number and multiply it by the ratio from earlier. For this example, you would have to consume 89.6 grams of protein each day to preserve your muscle mass. It looks like this:

$$112 \text{ pounds muscle} \times 0.8 \text{ grams protein} = 89.6 \text{ grams}$$

Our last macro is fats. We must consume an adequate amount of fats to maintain cell membranes, provide protective cushioning for organs, absorb certain vitamins, and promote development, growth, and energy. These fats will also help you stay full.

Dietary fat is broken down into glycerol and fatty acids. The body can't synthesize two types of fatty acids, so it's important that you consume them in your diet. These fatty acids are linolenic acid and linoleic acid.

These fats are sating, so they're perfect for people looking to fight off hunger pangs. Now you must figure out how much fat you need to eat. If your carbs are at a minimum, you've figured out how much protein you need to eat. You must meet the rest of your dietary needs with fats.

To maintain weight, you will eat enough calories from fats to support your regular expenditure. If you want to burn fats, you will have to eat in a deficit.

I have given you a lot of information to help you figure out your macros. However, there is an easier way to figure this out. Many online calculators are available to calculate these numbers without giving you a headache. If you want to use an online calculator, check out the website Ketogains. It has a calculator that works well.

If you want to see how figuring it out on your own will work, let's continue with the 160-pound example from earlier. Let's say this person is a female, stands 5'4", is in her late 20s, and has a desk job. She's mainly sedentary.

Plugging her information into a calculator:

The base metabolic rate would be 1,467 kcal.

The daily energy expenditure would be 1,614 kcal.

She would need to eat around 90 grams of protein, 20 grams of net carbs, and 86 grams of fat. Her intake is made up of 72 percent fat, 23 percent protein, and 5 percent carbs.

Now you know what macros are and how to figure out your numbers. You are well on your way to starting on a ketogenic diet.

The Dark Side of Keto

While the keto diet, for the most part, is a safe and effective diet, it does have some downsides and dangers. Before we look at the dangers, let's look at the side effects you may experience once you have entered ketosis.

Not all these keto side effects are bad, but a few are definitely unpleasant.

1. You could feel sick and tired.

The keto flu is real. When you cut your carbs and reach ketosis, you will experience a number of uncomfortable symptoms, such as diarrhea, nausea, muscle aches, fatigue, and headaches. These side effects are caused by the body's transition to using fat as its main energy source instead of carbs. Once your body has adapted to this fuel source, after about a week or two, you will feel a lot better.

1. Weight will drop quickly, but some could come back.

Keto diets are popular because of the initial quick slim down. This is because your body will release a lot of water when it starts using fat for energy. The scales will probably go down a few pounds, and you may even appear leaner.

That first drop you experience is likely only water weight. That doesn't mean you haven't burned off any fat, though. The problem is, while studies have found that you will lose weight, they haven't figured out whether this loss is sustainable in the long term. Most people will find the strict eating plan tough to stick to. If you end up veering off the diet, you could gain back all that weight.

1. You could feel less hungry.

Most diets are associated with fighting off cravings and feeling hungry. That's not necessarily the case with the keto diet. Many people report less hunger and a diminished need for eating. Researchers aren't completely sure why this happens, but it's believed that low-carb diets suppress the hormone ghrelin, which controls hunger.

1. You will be thirstier.

Don't be worried when you start feeling more parched on a keto diet. You will be excreting a lot of water, which will spike your thirst. Drink plenty of water. There isn't an exact amount, but you should drink enough to turn your urine from pale yellow to clear.

———————

1. Your skin could clear up.

IF PIMPLES HAVE BEEN bothering you, the keto diet could clear them up. This is especially true if you used to be a sugar addict. Empty carbs are the worst thing for acne because they trigger inflammation. Some studies have found that curbing your carb intake could fix those types of problems.

1. You might have less brain fog.

Everybody knows that carbs – especially the refined kind, like white pasta, white bread, and sugar – cause blood sugar spikes and dips. So, it's easy to see why eating fewer of them will keep your blood sugar steady. If you are healthy, this means you will have steady energy, fewer sugar cravings, and less brain fog.

1. It could mean better A1C levels.

If you are diabetic, the better blood sugar control could help control your A1C. It might even reduce your need for insulin. That doesn't mean you should go off your meds, though. The only caveat is that it also increases your risk of diabetic ketoacidosis, which is life-threatening. This is more common among people with type 1 diabetes, but if you have type 2, you should still talk to your doctor first.

1. You might experience low energy levels.

This is a common feeling as your body is adjusting to your fuel source switch. Luckily, once your body has adjusted, your energy levels will increase.

The Dangers of Keto

We've talked about the side effects that the keto diet can cause. The negative ones will typically go away once your body has adjusted to the diet. Following are some not-necessarily-temporary things that could happen to you on the keto diet. These are rare, but they could happen.

1.   Low blood sugar

For the most part, once you have reached ketosis, you will notice more stable and lower blood sugar levels. That's why low-carb diets are effective at controlling type 2 diabetes. Carb monitoring has been used for a while as a way to control blood sugar. However, one study has found that low-carb diets aren't better for long-term control than any other diet.

Some anecdotal evidence indicates that people with type 2 diabetes were able to stop taking their medicine because they had stabilized their blood sugar. However, that is not recommended. People with diabetes must talk to their doctors first.

During those first few days, when the body is still adapting to the changes, your body is in a constant struggle. If you have diabetes, you must ease your way into the diet. Slowly cut back on your carbs. Otherwise, you could cause your blood sugar to drop too much.

1.   Nutritional deficiencies

A high-fat, low-carb diet will limit the kinds of foods you are able to eat, and will eliminate entire food groups. Whole grains, beans, and legumes are all out, as are many vegetables and fruits. Most of these foods carry nutrients, vitamins, and minerals you can't get anywhere else. Without those foods, you could experience nutritional deficiencies.

Keto isn't good for a long-term diet because it's not balanced. Diets devoid of veggies and fruits will cause long-term micronutrient deficiencies that will create other consequences. They are great for short-term fat loss, but are best followed under the supervision of a medical professional.

1. Constipation and bowel changes

Eliminating veggies and fruits causes problems other than a lack of nutrients. These are fiber-rich foods that help you regulate your bowels. Without them, you may experience bowel changes, including difficulty having bowel movements and possible constipation.

To help prevent this, load up on fiber-rich, low-carb foods like cabbage, asparagus, and broccoli as well as more fats like ghee and coconut oil.

1. Loss of electrolytes

When you hit ketosis, your body will start dumping stores of glycogen, which is found in your muscles, and fat that carries extra weight. This will cause you to use the bathroom more and will lead to electrolyte loss. Electrolytes are important for proper cardiac function and normal heartbeats. This could cause a cardiac arrhythmia.

Try to get more electrolytes through natural sources or OTC supplements.

1. Decreased serum sodium

The average American consumes way too much salt. However, a person on keto can struggle to get enough. Low sodium levels can cause confusion, decreased energy, leg cramps, and vomiting. Make sure that you add salt to all your meals. Sea salt is the best because it contains trace minerals.

1. Dehydration

This is more common among people who are just starting keto because ketosis will flush water from your body. To help prevent dehydration, aim to consume

2.5 liters of water each day, as soon as you start this diet. Don't wait until you notice the ill effects.

1.   Kidney damage and kidney stones

If you don't take control of dehydration, it can lead to acute kidney injury. However, that's not the only way you could end up hurting your kidneys with a keto diet. Excess protein can create high nitrogen levels, which increase pressure in the kidneys. This can cause kidney stones and damage your kidney cells.

1.   Muscle loss

The longer your body stays in ketosis, the more fats it will burn. However, you could lose muscle tissue as well. While protein is the powerhouse and does a lot for building muscle, your muscles also need carbs for maintenance and formation. Without carbs, the body could break down your muscles.

1.   Cardiac problems

Losing some heart muscle isn't the only heart-associated risk that could accompany the keto diet. If you are already on medication for high blood pressure, and if you are on the keto diet, you could end up with abnormally low blood pressure. If you already have a heart condition, talk to your doctor before you start a keto diet.

Why You Should Try Keto

———

———

I KNOW YOU JUST FINISHED reading a chapter about the side effects and dangers associated with the ketogenic diet. You may be a bit apprehensive. However, this chapter will describe all the good things it can do.

Lots of amazing things can happen when you follow a ketogenic diet. Let's discuss a few.

Focuses the Brain

The keto diet can help increase memory, clarity, cognition, and seizure control, and lessen migraines. The first notable use of the ketogenic diet was in the 1920s at the Mayo Clinic, to help children with epilepsy. While the exact reason why seizure prevention occurs on a keto diet is still unknown, scientists think it's because the keto diet causes an increased stability of neurons and up-regulation of mitochondrial enzymes and brain mitochondria.

Similarly, the diet's effects on Alzheimer's disease have received a significant amount of attention. Researchers have discovered an increase in cognition and improved memory in adults who experience problems in these areas. Additional research has found improvement in all dementia stages. Ketosis can also help fight Parkinson's disease.

The wider audience of keto diet followers has reported side effects including a decrease in the intensity and frequency of migraines as well as better mental focus and clarity. This is likely due to the more stable blood sugar and change in brain chemistry that promotes cognition and memory.

Fights Cancer

Dom D'Agostino's lab found that ketone supplementation decreased the viability of tumor cells and prolonged the lives of mice that had metastatic cancer.

Cancer cell metabolism worked abnormally compared to healthy cell metabolism. Cancer cells increase glucose consumption because of mitochondrial dysfunction and genetic mutations. Some studies have found that, unlike healthy tissues, cancer cells can't effectively use ketone bodies for energy. Ketones will also inhibit the viability and proliferation of tumor cells.

This doesn't mean a cancer patient should forgo regular treatment. Be sure to follow your doctor's advice.

Prevents Heart Disease

A keto diet can lower triglycerides and blood pressure as well as improve cholesterol profiles. This is because the keto diet keeps blood glucose stable and low. While it may sound counterintuitive that eating more fat will lower triglycerides, excess carb consumption is, in fact, the main driver of high triglycerides.

A keto diet helps increase levels of HDL (i.e., the good cholesterol) and improves LDL profiles.

Decreases Inflammation

A *Nature Medicine* article reported that a keto diet is anti-inflammatory in nature and can help with a host of related issues.

Research has found that these effects could be connected to "BHB-mediate inhibition of the NLRP3 inflammasome."

Basically, inflammatory diseases can be suppressed by BHB, which is a ketone produced when one is on a ketogenic diet. This has significant implications for IBS, eczema, psoriasis, acne, arthritis, and other inflammatory diseases, prompting more research attention.

Improves Sleep and Energy

Once people reach day four or five of the diet, many of them report an increase in energy levels and fewer cravings for carbs. Again, the main reason for this is the stable insulin levels and an energy source that is readily available for the brain and body tissues.

It's still a mystery as to why the keto diet helps improve sleep. However, some studies have found that a keto diet helps sleep because it decreases REM and increases slow-wave sleep patterns. The exact reason for this is unclear. It probably has to do with the complex biochemical shifts involved in the brain's use of ketones for energy combined with the body's burning of fat.

Promotes Stable Uric Acid Levels

One of the main causes of gout and kidney stones is elevated levels of uric acid, phosphorus, oxalate, and calcium. This is normally due to a combination of: the consumption of food and beverages with lots of alcohol and purines; sugar consumption; obesity; dehydration; and unlucky genetics.

There is a caveat, though. A ketogenic diet will temporarily raise uric acid levels, especially if you allow yourself to become dehydrated. However, over time, the levels will decrease.

Promotes Gallbladder and Gastrointestinal Health

This means you will experience less bloating and gas, improved digestion, less risk of gallstones, less acid reflux, and less heartburn.

Sugary foods, nightshades (like tomatoes and potatoes), and grain-based foods increase a person's likelihood of experiencing heartburn and acid reflux. Therefore, it shouldn't come as a surprise that eating a few carbs will improve these symptoms and confront the root problems of autoimmune responses, inflammation, and bacterial issues.

A keto diet will also reproducibly and rapidly alter the human gut microbiome. Dr. Eric Westman has explained that these microbiome changes can eliminate or reduce a large number of problems.

In addition, research has found that carb consumption is one of the main causes of gallstones. When you consume enough fat while your carb intake is down, you will help clear up your gallbladder and make things run more smoothly.

Promotes Women's Health

A review published in 2013 looked at how a keto diet can enhance fertility. Research has found that PCOS can be effectively treated with a low-carb diet which will reduce or eliminate symptoms like obesity, acne, and prolonged or infrequent periods.

Overall, keeping your blood sugar stable and low will help stabilize and equilibrate other hormone levels. This will naturally cause downstream benefits in a wide array of metabolic pathways related to insulin, like energy utilization and hunger.

Helps Eyes

One of the biggest problems diabetics can face is macular degeneration. High blood sugar can hurt a person's eyesight and lead to a greater risk of cataracts. When you keep your blood sugar levels low, you will improve your vision.

Improves Endurance and Helps You Gain Muscle

BHB has been found to promote muscle gain. This fact, combined with tons of anecdotal evidence from over the years, has created a bodybuilder movement towards adopting a keto approach to gaining muscle.

Ultra-endurance athletes have also turned to the keto diet. Evidence suggests that once an athlete has become fully fat-adapted, their physical and mental performance improves.

Improves Metabolic Syndrome, Diabetes, and Obesity

This is the biggest reason why people start a ketogenic diet. For pretty much every reason we have covered, a keto diet is great for people who have type 1 or type 2 diabetes.

It is also extremely effective for obesity in that it helps burn fat and spares muscle loss. It also curbs disorders related to obesity. This includes all the risk factors and symptoms known as metabolic syndrome.

Different Types of Ketogenic Diets

⸺

You know all the positive and negative things that can happen when you follow a ketogenic diet. Now you must decide which diet will work for you. Yes, there is more than one keto diet. To get the most from it, you should pick the diet that works best for your needs and health goals. Each type works better for different types of lifestyles.

The Four Keto Types

There are four types of ketogenic diets that you can follow depending on your goals.

If you lead an active life or are an athlete who practices high-intensity training, one of these keto diets is perfect for you. If you want to simply lose fat and reach your best health, one of these is perfect for you, too.

1. The standard ketogenic diet – therapeutic and fat loss purposes.
2. Targeted ketogenic diet – workout performance.
3. Cyclical ketogenic diet – athletes and bodybuilders.
4. High-protein ketogenic diet – high-protein needs.

Each of these diets comes with its own rules. They will also differ in the number of net carbs you should eat each day.

Standard Ketogenic Diet

This option is best for beginners, anybody who wants to lose body fat, and people who want to follow it for therapeutic and insulin resistance purposes.

You will start by eating 20 or fewer net carbs per day. The rest of your diet is made up of 75 percent fats and 20 to 25 percent protein.

This is the most common type of ketogenic diet and is probably the best version to start with if you have never followed a keto diet before. This is the diet that is most commonly used to describe the keto diet and it works best for a vast majority of people.

The standard diet's rules are:

- 20 grams of net carbs each day. Some resources will say that you can eat up to 50 grams of carbs, but to reach ketosis, you must eat 30 grams or fewer.
- An adequate amount of protein – 0.8 grams per pound of lean mass.
- A high amount of fat intake.

Targeted Ketogenic Diet

This is best for people who know their bodies well when in ketosis and for people who want to gain extra energy for their workouts.

Your net carb intake will be around 20 to 50 grams fewer every day, normally 30 minutes to an hour before exercising. This is a good idea for athletes who are active.

This form of the keto diet is targeted specifically for workout energy. "Targeted" refers to eating immediately after or before your workout times. This form of keto is best for people who already know their limits and want to push themselves out of ketosis. This is ideal if you want to maintain exercise performance and let glycogen re-synthesis happen without interrupting ketosis.

When you follow a targeted diet, you will need to consume 25 to 50 grams of net carbs an hour or so before you start your exercise. This is the number of carbs that will make up your day.

This is a diet best suited for people who don't need to carb load, such as those who follow a cyclical ketogenic diet and those who don't want to exert the energy needed to optimize a cyclical diet.

The best types of carbs for a targeted diet are high-glycemic-index because they are easily digestible. You want to aim for foods that are high in glucose. Stay away from fructose. Fructose will give the liver the glycogen it needs instead of creating muscle glycogen, which is what a keto diet tries to avoid.

This will help prevent the disruption of ketosis because you will burn the carbs effectively and quickly during your training sessions. If you are consuming most of your carbs around the time you work out, you must watch out for your hidden carbs.

Both targeted and cyclical diets are used for high-intensity exercise, but just because you are an athlete or have an active lifestyle doesn't mean you must follow either one of these keto types.

Extra carb consumption has long been recommended for people who are active and who perform high-intensity exercise regularly. However, some recent research shows that this isn't necessarily the case.

Cyclical Ketogenic Diet

This is the best choice for athletes, bodybuilders, and those who have followed a keto diet before.

For this diet, you will consume a low number of net carbs five to six days a week. You will consume a higher carb diet for the remaining one to two days in the week. Then this cycle will repeat. People who must have carbs should follow this diet.

The cyclical diet works similarly to the idea of intermittent fasting, which is followed by the 5/2 style of fasting, because of its up and down days. The cyclical diet involves eating a keto diet for most days of the week and is followed by a day or two of high carbs. These days are referred to as "carb-loading."

Carb-loading involves alternating days on a keto diet with high-carb-consumption days. These high-carbs days could be 24 to 48 hours long. Normally, a cyclical diet requires that you consume around 50 grams of net carbs every day during the first phase, then around 450 to 600 grams of net carbs during the last phase.

Just like a targeted diet, a cyclical diet is best for people who understand their limits and cannot break through their boundaries without some carbohydrate consumption.

This is best for bodybuilders and athletes who want to maximize fat loss while building their lean muscle mass.

The advanced athlete who performs high-intensity and high-volume exercises would reap the most advantages from this keto diet. The goal of cyclical is to deplete your muscle glycogen between your carb loads, while a targeted diet keeps your muscle glycogen at a moderate level.

High-Protein Ketogenic Diet

This is best for people who want to follow the standard diet but need or want to consume more protein.

This works almost exactly like the standard ketogenic diet, except you consume more grams of protein each day. This means that instead of consuming five percent carbs, 70 percent fats, and 25 percent protein, you would eat five percent carbs, 60 percent fats, and 35 percent protein. This is great for people who lift four to six days a week.

While you will be consuming more protein in this diet, it won't be enough to cause your blood sugar levels to increase and knock you out of ketosis. A big myth about the keto diet is that if you eat too much protein, you will be knocked out of ketosis due to gluconeogenesis.

The process of GNG is extremely stable. You can't easily change the rate of GNG even when you eat extra protein. GNG is the process of creating glucose from non-carbs, but it doesn't work at the rate as carb metabolism.

When a person consumes chocolate cake, their blood glucose spikes because they consumed sugar during a very small window of time. When a person eats extra protein, the blood glucose won't spike because GNG will remain stable.

Muscle Maintenance

Are you worried about muscle loss on the keto diet? Your body has some mechanisms that will contribute to muscle growth and maintenance while you're on a keto diet.

The ketones that the liver produces for energy contain protein-sparing proper-ties which will prevent your muscles from breaking down. This is beta-hydrox-ybutyrate, BHB.

Adrenaline also plays a role in preserving muscle when in ketosis. When your blood sugar drops, your body will send out a signal for the production of adren-al secretion. This secretion helps regular muscle mass through adrenergic influ-ences.

This means that when the blood glucose drops because of a decrease in carb in-take, the body will send a signal to the adrenal gland, telling it to release epi-nephrine. Muscle proteins are greatly affected by these types of influences be-cause of their hormonal activity, which inhibits muscle breakdown.

This brings us back to the high-protein diet. As you know, on this diet you will consume more protein than is typically recommended for ketosis. When you consume an adequate amount of protein, you will maintain muscle mass.

While it may appear that you are consuming low amounts of protein, keep in mind that once your body is keto-adapted, it will utilize ketones and fats for energy, which will let it depend on these sources (instead of protein) for fuel.

How to Pick a Diet

I can't give you a straightforward answer to this. The "calories in versus calories out" rule works only to an extent. This rule doesn't consider what you are burn-ing – either lean mass or body fat.

While it may seem simple (meaning it doesn't matter what you are eating as long as you expend more than you take in), a number of other variables haven't been put into play.

Yes, you will lose weight when you eat a caloric deficit, but some of the weight loss will come from muscles. Research has found that while you consume only 15 to 25 percent of protein on keto, you can eat a caloric deficit in ketosis with-out burning muscle mass.

If you are a complete beginner, it is best to start with a standard ketogenic diet. This will allow your body to adjust quickly and make the transition into ketosis easier.

Even if you live an active lifestyle, or if you're an athlete, beginning with SKD will guarantee a change of metabolism so that you won't have to wonder whether you've hit ketosis.

Once you have brought up your ketone level, adding some carb-loading days could be an option. Don't use these carb-loading days as cheat days. You must be careful because any of these high-carb days could end up kicking you out of ketosis. Then you might need a week to get back into ketosis.

Reaching Ketosis

I'VE THROWN AROUND "ketosis" a few times in this book. Let's talk about what exactly it is. Ketosis is a natural state that the body enters when fat is fueling it. This happens when a person fasts or follows a strict low-carb diet.

Ketosis has several possible benefits, such as performance, health, and weight loss. However, as we have talked about in the "dangers" chapter, it comes with side effects. In people who have type 1 diabetes and other diseases, excessive ketosis could be dangerous.

When in ketosis, the body produces ketones. These are small fuel molecules which the body uses as an alternative fuel source when glucose is in short supply. The liver will start converting fat into ketones that are released into the bloodstream. The body will use these just like glucose. Ketones can also fuel the brain.

Hitting Ketosis

There are two ways your body can reach ketosis: a ketogenic diet or fasting. Under either one of these circumstances, once the body's limited amount of glucose has been depleted, the body will switch its source of fuel to fat. Levels of the fat-storing hormone insulin will become low, and the body's fat burning will increase. This means your body has easy access to your fat stores and can get rid of them.

You are considered to be in ketosis once your body produces enough ketones to constitute a significant level in the blood, usually more than .5mM. The quickest way for this to happen is through fasting, but this isn't something you can do forever.

That's why people turn to a keto diet, as it can be followed for an indefinite amount of time.

Brain Fuel

Many people think you must have carbs to fuel your brain. The brain will happily burn carbs when you consume them, but when carbs aren't available, it will eat ketones.

This is necessary for basic survival. Because the body is able to store carbs for only a day or two, the brain would end up shutting down after a few days with no food. Alternatively, just to keep working, it would need to quickly convert muscle protein into glucose, which isn't very efficient. That would mean we could waste away very quickly. If this were the way the body worked, the human race wouldn't have been able to survive before 24/7 food became available.

The body has evolved to work smarter than that. Normally, the body has fat stores that will last, so that a person can survive for several weeks without food. Ketosis is the process that ensures the brain is able to run on those fat stores.

Ketosis and Ketoacidosis

Many misconceptions surround ketosis. The main one is to confuse it for ketoacidosis, which is a rare and dangerous condition that typically occurs only among people who have type 1 diabetes. Even some health care professionals will mix up these two things, perhaps because the names are similar and there is a lack of knowledge about the distinct differences.

Ketosis is a natural state during which the body is in complete control of itself. Ketoacidosis is a malfunction in which the body creates an unregulated and excessive amount of ketones. This will cause symptoms like stomach pain, nausea, and vomiting, which are then followed by confusion and a coma. This will require urgent medical treatment and could be fatal.

Ketoacidosis occurs when ketones reach levels of 10 millimolar or more. People who follow a keto diet normally reach levels of three millimolar or less. Many people struggle to reach 0.5 millimolar. Long-term starvation, which means you have gone without food for a week or longer, could bring the number to six or seven. Ketoacidosis can happen at level 10, but more commonly happens at 15 plus.

The difference between these processes is like drinking a glass of water versus drowning in the ocean. Both deal with water, but they are far from the same thing.

If your pancreas functions properly and produces insulin, meaning you don't have type 1 diabetes, it would be very hard for you to hit ketoacidosis, even if you wanted to. The reason for this is that, when it produces too many ketones, your body will release insulin. This will shut down ketone production.

Reaching Optimal Ketosis

This is what everybody on a ketogenic diet wants. When you reach optimal ketosis, your body burns fat at the most optimal speed. To reach this optimal ketosis, you must follow the low-carb, high-fat diet as laid out above, keeping your macros in the optimal range. There isn't any trick to help you reach this optimal level. However, you can do certain things.

Here are the different ketone levels you could achieve:

- Below 0.5 means you are not in ketosis.
- Between 0.5 and 1.5 is a light level of nutritional ketosis. You will be losing weight, but it won't be optimal.
- Around 1.5 to 3 is considered optimal ketosis and is best for maximum weight loss.
- Levels over 3 aren't necessary. High levels won't help you and could end up harming you because they could mean that you aren't getting enough food.

Many people believe they are consuming a strict keto diet but end up being surprised when they measure their blood ketone levels. They end up being around 0.2 or 0.5, which isn't at that sweet spot.

The trick to get past this plateau is to not only avoid the obvious carb sources but make sure your protein intake isn't higher than your fat intake. I know I said that protein won't affect your glucose levels as easily as carbs do, but if you consume too much protein, especially if you eat more of it than fat, your glucose will be affected. This will compromise your optimal ketosis.

The secret to working around this problem involves your intake of fat. Add a big dollop of herbed butter to your steak. This could prevent you from eating as much or going back for seconds.

A glass of bulletproof coffee can also help stave off hunger and prevent you from eating too much protein. This is as easy as adding a tablespoon of butter and a tablespoon of coconut oil to your coffee in the morning.

The more fats you eat, the fuller you will feel. This will ensure that you don't eat too much protein and that you eat fewer carbohydrates. This should help you reach optimal ketosis.

Measuring Ketosis

There are a few ways to figure out whether you have reached ketosis. The first way is to measure the ketones in your blood. This requires purchasing a meter and will require a prick of the finger.

Quite a few reasonably priced gadgets are out there for this purpose, and it takes only a few seconds to determine your blood ketone level. Most people don't go to this extreme to find out what their ketone level is, but it is the most accurate and effective method.

Measure your blood ketones first thing in the morning, on a fasted stomach. Follow the levels that I listed earlier in this chapter to figure out if you are in ketosis.

These meters measure the amount of BHB in your blood. This is the main ketone that will be present when you are in ketosis. This method's main downside is the fact that you must draw blood.

A test kit will cost around $30 to $40, and could cost an extra $5 for every test. This is the reason why those who choose to test this way will perform only one test every week or every other week.

If you don't want to take on the expense of getting a blood ketone meter, here are nine other methods to figure out whether you are in ketosis.

1. Bad breath

This doesn't sound pleasant, but people often say they have bad breath when they hit ketosis. This is a fairly common side effect. People say their breath becomes fruitier.

The reason for this is the elevated ketone levels. The main culprit is the ketone acetone, which the body excretes through your breath and urine. While you may not like the idea of having bad breath, it is a great way to determine whether you're in ketosis. Many people will brush their teeth more often or chew sugar-free gum.

1. Weight loss

This is probably the most obvious way to know whether you're in ketosis. When you first start a keto diet, you will experience a fast drop in weight. However, this is typically water weight. The next drop in weight you'll experience will be your fat stores. This is how you will know that you are in ketosis.

1. Ketones in urine and breath

If you don't want to prick your finger, you can measure blood ketones using a breath analyzer. This will monitor for acetone, which is one of the three ketones present in your blood once you reach ketosis.

The measurement will let you know when your ketone levels have hit ketosis level because acetone will leave the body only once you reach nutritional ketosis. These breath analyzers are fairly accurate, though not as accurate as a blood monitor.

Another way to check for ketosis is to use special indicator strips to test for ketones in your urine every day. This is a quick and cheap method of assessing your ketone levels every day. These aren't the most reliable methods, though.

1. Appetite suppression

Many people report that their hunger decreases when they follow a ketogenic diet. The main reasons for this are still under study. However, it's believed that the reduction in hunger is due to an increase in vegetable and protein consumption as well as a change to your hunger hormones. The ketones may also affect the way your brain reacts to hunger.

1. Better energy and focus

Many people report feeling sick or tired or having brain fog when they first start a keto diet. This is the keto flu, but people who follow the diet long term will report more energy and increased focus. Your body must take the time to adapt to the new diet. Once you hit ketosis, your brain will start burning ketones for energy. This could take a week or so to start happening.

Ketones are a more potent fuel source for the brain than are carbs. This means ketones will improve your mental clarity and brain function.

1. Short-term fatigue

When your body is making the initial switch to keto, you might experience fatigue and weakness, which can make it hard for some people to stick with the diet. This is a natural side effect, but it lets you know that you are hitting ketosis.

This initial crappy feeling can last for a week to a month before you hit full-on ketosis. To help reduce this feeling, take an electrolyte supplement.

1. Short-term performance decrease

Just like with number six, fatigue can cause a decrease in exercise performance. This is due to the reduction in your muscle glycogen stores, which is what typically provides you with the fuel you need for high-intensity exercises. After a week or so, your performance levels should return to normal.

1. Digestive issues

With the major changes to the foods you eat, you will probably initially experience diarrhea or constipation. This lets you know that you are reaching ketosis. After your transition period, these issues should go away.

1. Insomnia

One of the biggest issues a keto dieter will have is insomnia, especially when they first start. When a person's carbs are drastically reduced, sleeping issues can result. However, this too shall pass.

Many different signs and symptoms will let you know whether you are in ketosis, and whether you are doing things correctly. Ultimately, if you follow the rules for a keto diet and keep yourself consistent, your body will be in some form of ketosis.

The only way to know for certain whether you are in ketosis is with a blood ketone monitor.

Exercising While Ketogenic

WHEN YOU EXERCISE MORE often, your health will improve. If you follow a keto diet, you will lose weight rapidly and improve your health. However, what happens if you combine the two?

It would be a reasonable assumption that combining the two would take your weight loss and health to the next level. However, the truth is a touch more complicated. With your new restriction of carbs, a plethora of changes will occur, some of which will affect your exercise performance.

With your restricted intake of carbs, you prevent your muscle cells from getting sugar, which is the fastest fuel source. When muscles aren't able to access sugar, their high-intensity function is impaired. "High-intensity" refers to any activity lasting longer than 10 seconds. The reason for this is that after 10 seconds of almost maximum effort, the muscles will start turning to glucose for energy through a metabolic pathway known as glycolysis instead of the phosaphen system.

During this time, fat and ketones aren't good substitutes for glucose. Only after you have been exercising for about two minutes will your body shift into a metabolic pathway capable of using your fat and ketones.

Basically, when you restrict your carb intake, you are depriving your muscles' cells of sugar, which they need to fuel activities for high-intensity effort from 10 seconds to two minutes. This means if you are on a ketogenic diet, it will limit your performance during exercises like:

- Weight lifting for more than five reps, each set using a weight heavy enough to bring you close to failure.
- Swimming or sprinting for over 10 seconds.
- Playing a sport that gives you minimal breaks such as lacrosse, rugby,

or soccer.
- High-intensity circuit training or interval training.

This is by no means comprehensive, but it does give you a decent idea of the kinds of exercises for which your body must use glycolysis. Remember, though, that the metabolic pathway timing will depend on each person. Some people can maintain performance for 30 seconds without needing carbs.

It's also important to consume the right amount of protein and fat when you are exercising on keto.

Most health professionals, when designing a diet plan, will set the protein intake first. Protein gets the top priority because it performs many actions that fats and carbs can't. Protein helps improve satiation, has a better thermic effect, and stimulates muscle synthesis better than any of the other macronutrients. Plus, if you don't consume enough protein, you will end up losing muscle mass and could end up consuming more calories.

If you plan to keep or implement your exercise regimen, which you should, you want to eat the right amount of macros. Here are a few guidelines:

- Keep your protein intake to a gram per pound of body weight.
- The majority of excess calories must come from fat, not from carbs or protein.
- Make sure your calorie intake stays around a deficit of 250 to 500 calories. This isn't of top priority. On a keto diet, most people don't worry about calories all that much.

Now that we have established the fact that you must be smart and careful when it comes to eating while exercise, let's look at the specifics.

Keto and Cardio

Luckily, most of us aren't athletes, so adding an exercise routine won't be too difficult. Cardio workouts won't require you to exercise at high intensities which require your body to burn glycogen and sugar for results. All you must do is bring up your heart rate and keep it there.

Because cardio has a low to moderate intensity, a ketogenic diet won't impair your performance. In fact, when in ketosis, you may realize that you are able to work out for a longer period of time without tiring.

To get the most from your workout, aim for moderate intensity. When you are aiming for moderate-intensity physical activity, you must get your heart rate to 50 to 70 percent of your maximum heart rate.

To estimate your maximum heart rate, start by subtracting your age from 220. If you were a 50-year-old person, to figure out your age-related heart rate, you would take 220 and subtract 50. That gives you 170 beats per minutes. Then you could figure out the 50 percent to 70 percent levels, which would be:

- 70 percent – 170 x 0.70 = 119
- 50 percent – 170 x 0.50 = 85

This means a 50-year-old person, to participate in moderate-intensity physical activity, would need to keep their heart rate between 85 and 119 beats per minute.

While you are adapting to a ketogenic diet, try to aim for the bottom end of that range. Once you have been on the diet for a couple of weeks, you will find that you can maintain a higher heart rate without the need for extra carbs.

If you are also new to working out and cardio, you will want to stick to 50 percent of your max heart rate for around ten to 15 minutes. You can start increasing the duration by five or so every week until you are able to work out for 30 to 45 minutes at 50 percent of your max heart rate. Once you have done this, you can begin increasing your intensity level each week until you have reached 70 percent of your max heart rate.

If you're not sure what works best for cardio workouts, here are some examples:

- Swimming
- Aerobic training classes
- Recreational sports
- Interval training classes

- Circuit training
- Running
- Cycling

Remember, though, that because of the carb restriction, these workouts could decrease your power and strength. If you are aiming only for a good cardiovascular workout, it's not important that you push yourself to the max for your power and strength.

This doesn't mean that you can't increase your power and strength while on a keto diet. To achieve this, just practice some mindful exercising.

Weight Lifting and Keto

You can increase muscle mass, power, and strength while following a ketogenic diet. The best thing is that you can improve all these things at the same time by using the same program.

Remember how I said earlier that without glucose, your body can last for only 10 seconds on high-intensity exercises? This means if you are a weightlifter, you can improve power and strength as well as muscle mass by doing sets that don't last any longer than 10 seconds.

This also means that a program requiring five or more sets of five or fewer reps for each exercise is perfect for people on a ketogenic diet.

Some recent research has found that lower reps can be helpful when it comes to hypertrophy, meaning your muscles don't need you to pump out eight to 12 reps in a row to grow bigger. What the muscles are looking for is the right volume (which depends on the person) and for your volume to increase each week.

This means you can build muscles without carbohydrates. Carbs may be needed for some high-intensity work, but a bodybuilder does not have to consume lots of carbs to see results.

Supplementing

Many no-carb supplements can boost your exercise performance while you are following a ketogenic workout. Here are some supplements that are keto-friendly:

1. Creatine

This is probably one of the most well-studied exercise supplements. It is an effective and safe way to enhance the body's phosphagen system. This is why creatine is best for explosive weightlifters and athletes.

Consuming five grams of creatine monohydrate powder each day is a great way to supplement for people looking to increase their muscle mass, power, and strength.

1. MCT (medium chain triglycerides)

MCTs, as we talked about earlier, are a form of saturated fats sent straight to the liver once they have been digested. The liver will use these fats for more ketones, which are then sent to cells that need the energy. MCTs are a great option for endurance athletes and cardio training.

It is recommended that you supplement with one to two tablespoons of MCT oil or powder before any endurance workouts to get an extra boost of energy.

1. Exogenous ketones

These types of ketones, much like ketone esters and ketone salts, can provide a person with an instant energy source. There is a downside, though. These supplements may end up lowering your liver's production of ketones. Therefore, it would be best to use these along with MCTs to boost your ketone production.

Much like MCTs, exogenous ketones are great for endurance and cardio training athletes. The important thing is to stay hydrated when you use these supplements because they do have a diuretic effect.

1. Caffeine

It's not surprising that caffeine is a great way to improve exercise performance because of its stimulatory effects. However, once you start taking caffeine on a consistent basis, you could find that you no longer get the same boost because of the way the body adapts to the habitual intake. Plus, caffeine will increase your cortisol levels, which will decrease your ketone production. It's best to experiment with other supplements and limit the amount of caffeine you consume.

1. Taurine

This is an organic acid that helps exercise performance. In fact, researchers have discovered that it works better to help exercise performance than does caffeine.

In a recent study, scientists looked at the effects that taurine and caffeine had on fatigue and power on all-out cycling sprints. The taurine supplement that was used by itself decreased fatigue and improved power more than the other two supplements did.

This has a big implication for bodybuilders and athletes who follow a keto diet because this study looked at the energy system that tends to be the most affected by carb restriction. According to the study, the participants took 50 mg of taurine per kilogram of weight. This would probably be a safe metric to use to figure out how much you should take. You could also slowly decrease the amount to see if you still get any effect.

1. Beta-alanine

This is a common compound in most pre-workout supplements. It will give your body a tingly sensation. Most people report that when they take beta-alanine, they are able to perform one or two reps more when they are training in sets of eight to 15.

This means that beta-alanine is probably a great supplement for keto dieters who need a better glycolytic pathway to help them through their training. High-intensity athletes and bodybuilders will get the most from this supplement.

With this supplement, timing doesn't really matter. Aim for two to five grams of beta-alanine along with five grams of creatine each day. If you don't enjoy the tingly sensation it gives you, take a gram of beta-alanine two to five times during the day.

1. L-citrulline

This is a common supplement for cardiovascular health and sports performance. Some studies have discovered that supplements of L-citrulline help improve endurance and reduce fatigue for anaerobic and aerobic prolonged exercise. This is a great supplement for nearly every active person except for those who rely on the phosphagen system, such as powerlifters and golfers. To boost your exercise endurance, take 6,000 to 8,000 mg about an hour before you work out.

1. Protein powder

While it is best to consume most of your protein from natural sources, protein powder is a good idea when you need help meeting your protein needs. This is also great if you follow a vegan keto diet.

Stick with complete protein powders such as collagen, whey, casein, or a mix of plant proteins. Stay away from BCAA and EAA supplements because you will receive more benefits from a complete protein powder.

Use this by adding 20 to 40 grams of protein powder to a smoothie, or you can consume it after you work out to help stimulate muscle synthesis without affecting your ketosis.

1. Alpha GPC

Choline is an important part of your nervous system. Whenever you move a muscle in your body, choline is needed to activate acetylcholine, a neurotransmitter that will send a chemical signal to your muscles and make them mobile. The best way to get more choline is by taking an alpha GPC supplement.

Research has found that 600 mg of alpha GPC can enhance your power output and secretion of growth hormone. This suggests that this choline supplement is great for weightlifters and athletes.

1. Fish oil

The omega 3 fatty acids EPA and DHA, found in fish oil, help boost your recovery and stimulate muscle synthesis. The AHA recommends that you consume one gram of these each day. You can do this using a fish oil supplement or by eating three ounces of salmon or sardines each day.

The goal is to reduce your soreness, which means you must aim for a six-gram dose spread throughout the day.

Keto and Exercise in Harmony

To mix these two things, you must make the right changes to your diet and workout program so that you don't cause any adverse reactions, especially if you participate in high-intensity workouts.

When you are trying to incorporate exercise to improve your health, you can experiment a bit more than an athlete can. In general, try lifting weights and doing some cardio training every week. Do cardio two to three times each week and lift weight two to three times each week. Avoid doing them both on the same day.

Keto Diet for Everyone

PEOPLE TEND TO SHY away from diets if they think those diets will be too hard to implement into their lives. The great thing about keto is that it's not hard to implement, and it should interfere with your life anyway. To help everybody feel like they can try a ketogenic diet, this chapter will look at eating on a budget, eating out, eating during the holidays, and more.

Keto on a Budget

Many people assume that eating keto will be expensive, but it doesn't have to be. You will increase your fat intake. Fats will make you feel fuller than carbs do, which means you will no longer eat snacks between your meals. Not eating a bunch of snacks can save you money.

Because your protein levels don't really have to change, you won't have to buy expensive meats. Here are some more money-saving tips:

- Keep things simple. Your meals don't need many different parts. The fewer ingredients you use, the less money you will spend. If you make a simple omelet and you drink water with it, you will spend around $3.50. A Big Mac costs about $5.
- Use fresh vegetables whenever they are in season. The rest of the year, you can buy frozen.
- You can normally get a better deal if you buy a whole chicken and cut it apart on your own. Keep the carcass as well. You can use this to make broth.
- Pay attention to the deals that your grocery store offers and stock up on these items, especially if you use them a lot.

Plan out your meals and your shopping list. This will ensure that you stay organized and buy only the things you need. Planning out your shopping lists is the best way to prevent unnecessary spending and impulse purchases.

When you are actually shopping, you can do a few things to save money:

- Get regular cheese. You don't have to buy specialty cheeses. Don't get pre-shredded; buy in bulk. Then you can shred the cheese yourself.
- Don't buy packaged coleslaw. You can make your own at home.
- Get simple meats and stay away from specialty. Cooked meat may make for a great quick meal but choose the less exotic types.
- Don't worry about kale that costs a fortune. Go for other leafy greens that are cheaper but just as nutritious.
- Quit getting nuts, especially macadamias, because they will add up.
- Choose almond meal over almond flour. It is cheaper and works just as well as almond flour in most recipes. You can also grind your own almonds.
- When avocados are out of season, don't buy them.
- Purchase frozen or canned fish instead of fresh, especially when it comes to salmon.

Get the best quality foods you are able to afford. Just because everybody says you should eat organic doesn't mean you must. If you can't afford it, don't get it. The important thing is that you make your meals at home from scratch. Organic or not, they will be healthier for you.

Also, when picking meats, go with the cheaper cuts and make sure you check out the bargain deals.

Cook all your meals at home. This is cheaper than eating out. Go with easier recipes and avoid the fancy keto recipes.

Traveling

An important part of any diet is maintaining it when you aren't home. The key to maintaining your diet is to plan things out. The following will help you maintain your diet when traveling.

- Know your macros

Before you go on vacation, make sure that you know your macros. Memorize them, or at least have a keto app on your phone that will help you track your macros.

- Travel evaluation

The next step is to evaluate how long your trip will be. An overnight trip is pretty easy to prepare for. You'll need some frozen meals, a cooler, and a microwave. A weeklong trip will change things drastically and cause some complications. Knowing what you will be up against is the important thing.

After you have figured out the location and length of your trip, start looking at the resources you will have at your disposal once there.

It's a good idea to try to book a place that comes with a kitchen, such as a place on Airbnb. If you must stay at a hotel, try to find a room at an extended-stay hotel. These types of places normally have more extensive cooking equipment than a regular hotel. This will increase your flexibility for meal prep. It would be great if you could find a place with a full-size freezer and refrigerator. Staying with friends and family is a great choice because you will have access to a kitchen.

Lastly, the method by which you are getting there is also important. If you are driving, you will have more flexibility than if you travel by plane. TSA restrictions can prevent you from bringing certain foods with you because they must be repacked and weigh less than three ounces.

- Food options

Now you must think about the foods you can take. Non-refrigerated foods are a great option. Beef jerky, canned chicken, tuna, and salmon are all great. So are canned protein shakes and olives. All your snack foods, like pepperoni, string cheese, and dried nuts, are great, too. If you like eggs, try hard boiling some to take along with you.

When it comes to refrigerated foods, unless your trip isn't far from home, you will want purchase perishables once you arrive. This is where having a refrigerator at your place is important.

When you arrive, go to the store and buy meats and cheese. Another option is to make your meals ahead of time and freeze them before your trip. Pack them in a cooler and get them in the freezer as soon as you arrive. Then, each morning, set your meals for the day in the fridge to thaw for later consumption.

- Restaurants

Many restaurants, including fast food places, offer low-carb options. If you want a burger, ask them to wrap it in lettuce, or at least leave off the bun. Going with meats like fish and steak will typically keep you low-carb. Stay away from fries as your side option. Also, avoid beans and rice. Go for roasted veggies, asparagus, and salads. If you have a Chipotle nearby, you can get a bowl without beans or rice and fill it with sour cream, guacamole, cheese, and meat.

Travelling doesn't have to mean that you must stop dieting. There are many ways to work around this, and it's not too hard as long as you plan ahead.

Keto While Dining Out

Did your friends invite you out? Are you afraid to go? Well, you don't have to be. You can have delicious foods no matter where you go.

- Get rid of the starch.

Get rid of the bread. Say no to pasta. Pass on the potatoes. Bounce the rice. Don't let temptations enter your plate; make sure you order your meal without starchy sides.

When you order an entrée, most places will allow you to substitute extra veggies or a side salad in place of the starchy side. When you get a burger or a sandwich, ask for it to be wrapped in lettuce instead in bread. If the restaurant isn't willing to make any substitutes, just eliminate the item completely.

If you get your plate and it comes with a starch, look at your options. If you know that you can leave it there and not eat it, go ahead. If you don't think you can handle the temptation, ask your waiter to replace it. If the place where you are dining is more casual, you can take care of things by placing the starch in the trash.

- Add good fats.

Restaurant meals tend to be low in fat, which makes it hard to feel full when you don't eat carbs. However, you can fix this in a number of ways. Ask for extra butter and melt it on your meat or veggies. Get a vinegar- and olive-oil-based dressing for your salad. Many restaurants will serve cheap veggie oils that are full of omega 6 fats. The more seasoned keto dieter will carry a small bottle of olive oil with them.

- Watch out for condiments and sauces.

Sauces such as Bearnaise contain mainly fats. Things like ketchup contain mainly carbs, and gravies could go either way. If you don't know about a sauce, ask what's in it and avoid it if it has flour or sugar. You can also ask the restaurant to put the sauce on the side so that you can decide how much you will add.

- Choose drinks wisely.

The best drinks to accompany your meal are coffee, unsweetened tea, sparkling water, and water. If you want an alcoholic beverage, choose dry wine, champagne, or spirits, either straight or with club soda.

- Dessert

If you're not hungry, go with a cup of coffee or tea as you wait for the others to finish. If you do feel hungry, see if the restaurant has a cheese plate or berries with whipped cream.

- Buffets

This is where things get tricky. Set some ground rules before you leave the table. Avoid all grains and starches and aim for protein, veggies, and fats. Find the smallest plate possible. You can go back for more if you don't get filled up the first time. Take your time eating. Talk to your friends and sip on your drink.

You Don't Like to Cook

Maybe you've come home late and don't want to cook. You unexpectedly find that you aren't prepared for keto. Or you just might not enjoy cooking. How do you stay keto when you don't want to – or can't – cook at home? Here are some options so that you can stay keto.

1. Coffee and Tea

The easiest thing to do is curb your appetite with tea or coffee. This works extra well if you add plenty of butter or heavy cream. It can ease you through to your next planned meal without your having to fix anything else.

1. Low-Carb Snacks

Fill your pantry with low-carb essentials so that you can create a platter of low-carb goodies when you feel hungry. Some things to keep on hand are:

- Healthy oils
- Mayonnaise
- Olives
- Full-fat yogurt
- Deli meat
- Pate
- Cream
- Frozen berries
- Nuts
- Avocado
- Beef jerky
- Pork rinds
- Cheeses

- Canned fish

1. Have Leftovers

When you do cook, make doubles or even triples of your meals. You can freeze the leftovers. That way, your meal will be waiting for you when you don't want to cook.

1. Minimal Cooking

Boiling an egg, frying up a steak, or buying an already-cooked chicken are great ideas. Add a pre-bagged salad, some cheeses, and mayonnaise, and you've got a good dinner. This can make your meal quick and easy and it won't feel like you have to do anything. You can also jazz up your salads with all the low-carb pantry foods we mentioned earlier.

1. Get a Slow Cooker

This is great if you don't like being over a hot stove, or if you know you'll get home late. Throw everything in the slow cooker first thing in the morning, set it, and forget it. You'll have a meal waiting for you that night.

1. Fast Intermittently

Is what you're feeling actual hunger? Learn your body and figure out your appetite. Eat only when you are really hungry. This works with the first suggestion as well. Drink water or coffee; you may find that you weren't really hungry.

Keto During the Holidays

Holidays will happen, and they are the hardest times of the year to maintain any type of diet. This is a time of couch surfing, excess consumption, and binging TV shows ... and that's fine. However, this doesn't mean that you have to stop keto. In fact, it's these times when you can reevaluate yourself and check on your keto life. Take a look at all the amazing progress you have made and learn to move past those anxiety-inducing moments. Here's how:

1. Keep a Keto-Positive Mind

What does it mean to have a keto-positive mind? View this like the Commandments of the Low-Carb Followers: Thou shalt not drool over thy neighbor's turkey sandwich, thou shalt not make friends feel bad for having fried, thou shalt not gloat, and so on. Yes, you are keto, but you are also a compassionate and awesome person. Keep yourself composed and stay keto.

1. Knowledge is Power

You can download tons of apps that will let you know what exactly is in the food you are about to eat. This means if you see some delicious cheeses making the rounds at a party, you don't have to feel bad for tasting a new brand. The trick to succeeding during the holidays is to know what you say yes to by making well-informed and smart decisions. MyFitnessPal is a great choice for meal tracking and finding out what's in food.

1. Create Clear Goals

The best way to stay on track is to come up with clear goals. Everybody's keto lifestyle is a little bit different. The rules you come up with must be based on your goals, which will end up determining your actions. If you're looking to drop excess fats, that's going to look different from the goals of somebody trying maintain or gain. A keto-warrior could have a five-point backup plan. The only best goals are your own goals.

1. Plan to Fail

What does it mean to plan to fail? This means you set the bar so high that even if you don't reach your goal, you will come in higher than your expectations. This is the best win-win, and it's easy. If you know that dessert is your weakness, make your own keto cheesecake and take it to the party. Now you will be able to have your cake and eat it too.

1. Don't Engage in a Debate

When you get into the keto lifestyle, you might find it tempting to convert others to your way of life. However, it's important to understand that not everybody wants to take the step, especially when it comes to the holidays. Your aunt may not understand the reason why you have bacon for every meal of the day, nor does she want to. The important thing is to make sure you are taking the steps you need to stay on track. You don't have to look out for the entire family.

1. Be Gracious and Have an Escape

This brings us to another point. The holidays tend to be hard for everybody. Lot of traveling – and lots of family time – await you, and everybody has to make sacrifices. That could mean you must choke down your mom's over-seasoned meatloaf, but do it with a smile on your face because it's the holidays. A small sacrifice isn't a big deal when you look at the grander scheme of things. You could also try to keep from visiting around mealtimes.

1. Plan Things Away from the Couch or Table

One easy way to stay keto is to change the way you see everything. Instead of waiting for people to invite you to a party, where you end up anxious about what foods they will have, make the plans yourself. Invite your family friends on a trip, a walk around town, or to see a show. Many free events take place around the holidays, and everybody will feel happier with some exercise.

1. Cheating is Fine, Just Set the Rules

A huge taboo for keto-land is cheating. When somebody breaks the rules and eats something they regret, they end up sitting around berating their self for weeks on end. Stop it. You are in charge of the rules, and you can change those rules. If you have a round of fries, it doesn't mean you have screwed up everything. If you don't take these slips so hard, it will be easier to get back on track.

1. Say Thank You

People will offer you all kinds of things. It's what the holidays are about. The best thing to do is say thank you, accept it, and then continue talking. Odds are they won't take notice that you didn't eat their fudge; however, if you say no, it could upset them. Repeat after me: "Awesome, thank you." Then take it and smile.

1. Keep Calm

The holidays come around only once a year, but you have keto for life. If you must take a few weeks off to enjoy all the lovely festivities, go ahead. If you feel like you need to up your gym time to compensate for some carb-eating, go for it. If you're a keto warrior, go and keto on. Nobody out there will judge you for trying to do your best during a crazy time of the year. Don't kill yourself over one too many cookies or a cup of apple cider. Get back on track and everything will be fine.

Cheating on Keto

In every diet, you hear people talk about cheat days, but can you have a cheat day on keto?

The truth is, no matter how you slice it, cheat meals are bad for you. The keto diet may be simple, but it's not always easy. There are a few grey areas, so we'll talk a little about what would happen if you chose to cheat on a meal.

You may know some people who follow a long-term low-carb diet and who schedule their cheat days at normal times, like once a month or on the weekends. This creates a healthy mindset, but things work slightly differently for keto.

Let's look at the effects that cheating has on a ketogenic diet.

1. It can pop you out of ketosis.

Because cheating could take you out of ketosis, especially if it's heavy on the carbs, you must make sure you are prepared for this. You can also test your ketones after you eat a "cheat meal" to see if you were actually knocked out. Some things may not affect your ketosis, but others do.

1.   It can affect fat adaptation.

The body is making many changes and will alter certain hormones and enzyme production so that it can burn fat for fuel. Regular cheat meals can prevent your body from doing this. You've done all this work to turn your body into a fat-burning machine. Are you willing to reverse this with too many carbs? Any weight gain you may experience later is water weight, but too much could negate the keto effects, especially if you have many cheat meals.

1.   Cheats can spike blood sugar.

Carb consumption can cause your blood sugar to spike, especially if you have diabetes. This is important to remember if you are diabetic, pre-diabetic, or sensitive to refined carbs and sugar.

1.   Cheating could create cravings.

Interrupting your body's adaptation to ketones for fuel will cause more cravings for junk food. You may find that once you bounce back to keto meals, you still suffer serious cravings for a while until you have adapted back to keto. For many people, what starts as a moderate cheat becomes a binge.

1.   You may feel the keto flu again.

Think about those days when you first started keto, felt lousy, and wanted to give up. Cheat days could cause you to go back through those days. Cheat days could also make you feel out of control and unstable because of the hard changes in the way you eat.

Now that you understand what could happen if you cheat on keto, let's look at how you can cheat the right way. Cheat meals have the advantage of keeping you from going crazy. Cheats are sometimes able to help you stay on a diet. Just because cheat days can get you off track doesn't mean you should get upset if you do end up slipping on one meal. Forgive yourself and move on.

If you feel like you would do better by incorporating cheat meals, following are some of the best ways to do so:

1. Follow a Cyclical Diet

If you remember back to the chapter about the types of ketogenic diets, the CKD allows you to eat keto for five days a week; then you can eat more carbs the other two days. This diet can make sticking to keto more manageable.

1. Conscious Cheating

When you want a cheat meal, pick something that is worth it. This means to choose something you really enjoy – something that will satisfy you and allow you to eat mindfully. This will reduce the odds that you will binge. Another thing to try is finding a keto alternative for your favorite foods.

Ultimately, it's your choice as to whether you want to make cheat meals a normal part of your diet. Make sure you are prepared for any consequences. However, scheduling cheats could keep you from slipping.

Should You Follow Keto?

THE KETO DIET GETS a lot of praise for being a great weight-loss plan. However, the high-fat, low-carb life might not be for you.

By now. you have probably read articles or another book about this diet. It might seem like just another fad that won't last, but this diet has been around for over 100 years. This diet offers many health benefits. Research has shown that this diet can help with lose weight, prevent obesity, improve alertness and cognition, improve metabolic and cardiovascular conditions, and treat epilepsy.

This happens because while in ketosis, our bodies go through many phases of metabolic and hormonal adaptations. They learn to use the new source of energy that they are getting from fat.

When the body doesn't have glucose available for fuel, these fatty acids become ketones that cross the blood-brain barrier, giving the muscles, heart, and brain more energy. This will minimize the excess fats in the body.

Just like with any diet, you must keep some safety issues in mind. The keto diet is not right for everybody. Here are some situations in which the keto diet might be dangerous and must be avoided:

Nursing or Pregnant

Not many studies have been done to investigate the side effects that the keto diet creates in pregnant women. Studies have shown that some side effects might include inadequate growth in children, constipation, hormonal changes, dehydration, anemia, nutrient deficiency, and weight loss.

Prolonged ketosis while pregnant has been shown to cause developmental problems in the baby. It can affect the development of babies' brains and increase the risk of defects like spina bifida.

Due to the risk of harm to the baby, doctors do not recommend this diet for pregnant women.

Similarly, not many studies exist about the keto diet's effects on nursing women. Most women who are either nursing or pregnant need more fiber and protein than women who aren't pregnant. Increased fiber supports fetal development and growth, improves mom's digestion, and gives both mom and baby the minerals and vitamins they need.

Because we don't know the exact effects of a keto diet on nursing moms, it is best to adopt a moderate carb intake that is safe for both the baby and the mom.

Medication That Can Cause Hypoglycemia

These medications could cause hypoglycemia:

- Glinides like repaglinide or nateglinide
- Sulphonylureas like tolbutamide, glipizide, glimepiride, gliclazide, and glibenclamide
- Insulin

These medications are designed to help the body increase insulin. This, in turn, will lower blood sugar.

If you follow a low-carb keto diet while taking these medicines, you could develop hypoglycemia. It is extremely important that you discuss this with your doctor so that you can work together to prevent the risk of hypoglycemia before you begin a keto diet.

Blood glucose tests will allow you to spot and possibly avoid developing hypoglycemia. You will need to test more often than you normally would while your body is adjusting to the change in its intake of carbs.

Blood Sugar Issues or Diabetes

Some people who try the keto diet will initially have problems with low blood sugar or hypoglycemia. This might be dangerous if you can't stabilize your blood sugar while taking diabetes medications.

Evidence shows that diabetes can be prevented or at least slowed down with exercise and a healthy diet. To be safe, people who have a history of prediabetes, diabetes, or hypoglycemia should not try the keto diet without first consulting their doctors.

Changes in diet and weight loss could require a change in the dose of diabetes medication. Don't follow any type of restrictive diet without your doctor's supervision.

Other Medication

Other medicines shouldn't cause any significant risk but might need to be looked at to ensure you still need it. Your doctor can tell you whether any changes to your dosage are necessary.

Your physician might also have to regulate blood pressure medicines because your blood pressure might drop on a keto diet.

Nutrient Deficiency or Being Underweight

In spite of its being a high-fat diet, the keto diet might lead to weight loss. This can happen quite suddenly. If you are currently underweight, have any mineral or vitamin deficiencies due to your not eating enough, or have had eating disorders in the past, this diet isn't for you.

If you have a low BMI and want to try the keto diet to improve your blood sugar level but don't want to lose weight, consult a dietitian or your doctor so that you can modify the diet to make it doesn't affect your weight.

If you lose weight fairly easily, a diet that includes complex carbs along with lots of proteins and healthy fats will be better for you.

If you have undergone gastric bypass surgery, the keto diet might be very dangerous because of the risk of nutrient deficiencies resulting from a lack of consumed calories.

Children

For many years, the keto diet has been used with children who suffer from seizures. This must be done under medical supervision.

There are several things to keep in mind before beginning a keto diet to make sure all the macronutrients are balanced and appropriate for children.

Consult a dietitian or doctor before starting any child on the keto diet.

Kidney Disease or Kidney Stones

Kidney stones are a side effect of the keto diet. If there is a history of any type of kidney disease, you absolutely must talk to your doctor before beginning the keto diet. Your doctor must check your creatinine/calcium ratio to make sure you aren't risking complications like nephrolithiasis, which is a condition in which the kidneys contain dangerous levels of calcium.

Gallstones or Gallbladder Removal

People who had gallstones were told to stay away from fat, but this isn't the case now. The NHS says that low-fat diets might cause gallstone growth.

If you already have gallstones, eating more fat might cause some gallstone pain. If you want to try the keto diet, you might need to go very slowly or try the diet after your gallstones have been dissolved or removed.

A study in 2014 showed that high-fat diets actually prevented the formation of gallstones. This might be a long-term benefit of the keto diet.

Many people who have had their gallbladders removed have successfully followed a keto diet without adverse side effects.

Enzyme Deficiency or Defect

While these are very rare disorders, two serious contraindications of the keto diet exist; they are called porphyria and pyruvate carboxylase deficiency. These conditions are caused by problems with the production of heme and lipid metabolism. Heme is found in hemoglobin, which carries oxygen out of the lungs and into the other parts of the body.

People with these disorders will experience deficiencies of some enzymes, which makes it hard for them to metabolize large amounts of free fatty acids. If you follow the keto diet and have these deficiencies or other types of beta oxidations defects, dangerous complications – like irregular heartbeats, mental changes, and nervous system deterioration – can result.

Free fatty acids build up, but the body can't use them for energy. This is the main reason why the condition is dangerous. People who have porphyria and pyruvate carboxylase deficiency need a steady supply of glucose to give their organs energy. If glucose isn't present because of a keto diet, some life-threatening problems can arise. This is called a catabolic crisis. If you have a family history of mitochondrial disorders or suspect that you have these conditions, you must be tested by your doctor before you even think about going on a keto diet.

Myths About Keto

————

You might have known about the keto diet but were afraid to try it because of rumors you heard. We will talk about some of the most famous myths we've heard about the keto diet.

Not everybody gets the "keto flu" and everyone will react to this diet differently. Factors such as your activity level, overall health, age, and gender will affect your metabolism, how well you adapt to ketosis, and your hormonal health. Let's take a look at these diet myths and discover the truth behind them.

Keto Is a High-Protein, High-Fat Diet.

Unlike the Atkins Diet or other low-carb diets, the keto diet isn't high in protein. Protein intake must be moderate because this lets you get into ketosis and stay there. Too much protein will cause some protein to be changed into glucose. This won't keep your glucose levels low.

You might be wondering how much protein you need. Typically, you'll want to get about 20 percent of your daily calories from protein, five percent from carbohydrates, and 75 percent from fat. A low-carb, high-protein diet might require you to get about 30 to 35 percent of your calories from protein.

You Will Only Lose Weight on This Diet.

This diet will help people lost weight and burn fat. If you don't want to lose weight, you can still follow the diet to maintain your weight or gain weight.

Could you really gain weight on this diet? It's possible if you don't do the diet the right way and never get into ketosis.

The low-carb, high-fat diet is controversial, as some people think you lose weight because of the low calorie intake. Others think it is because of the hormonal changes that the diet causes. Many experts agree that the type of diet someone follows doesn't matter. If your calorie intake exceeds your needs or activity level, you will gain weight instead of losing it.

If you are eating more calories than you need, even if they come from protein and healthy fats, you will see the number on your scale increase.

If you are not looking to lose weight, should you still follow a keto diet? The keto diet has many benefits that go far beyond weight loss. This diet can help your body normalize blood sugar, regulate hormone production, improve digestive health, improve cognitive function, and possibly reduce the risk of heart disease or diabetes.

There Isn't Any Science Behind the Diet.

This is so false, it's funny. As stated above, the keto diet can help manage health conditions like cancer, muscle loss, Alzheimer's disease, epilepsy, high blood pressure, dyslipidemia, type 2 diabetes, insulin resistance, and obesity.

You Can't Work Out While Doing Keto.

Exercising can help everybody, including those on a keto diet. You might not feel as energized when your body is transitioning into ketosis, but this feeling will abate as your body adjusts. Even during high-intensity workouts, your performance won't decline.

You do not need to stop working out while on the keto diet. You might have to modify your workouts a bit, though. If you can handle it, exercising while in ketosis will burn fat two to three times faster. It can also maintain blood glucose levels, and you will notice less fatigue with activity.

To help your body during workouts, consume enough calories, including those from fat. Also, let your body recover between tough workouts.

If you find yourself struggling while working out and having a hard time recovering, try eating more carbs just before you exercise. If you fast while on the keto diet, save your high-intensity workouts for times when you are more fueled up.

You Lose Muscle Mass.

This is so false. The keto diet can help you gain muscle. If you combine strength training with the keto diet, you can increase your strength and build muscle. The American Heart Association claimed that low-carb diets will cause you to lose muscle tissue. There aren't any physiological requirements for humans to eat carbs, and keto won't cause a person to lose muscle mass.

Will this diet work without exercising? Yes, it will lead to several improvements in a person's overall health. However, exercising can kick things up a notch in terms of health benefits and body composition.

Everybody Will Get Keto Flu.

Each person will react differently to the keto diet. This makes it hard to figure out what side effects you will experience, how severe those effects will be, and how long they will last. Some people might smoothly transition into ketosis. Others may deal with sleep problems, digestive problems, brain fog, and more fatigue for weeks after they get into ketosis.

These side effects are uncomfortable, but they usually go away in a week or two, so be patient. You can lessen these changes by drinking lots of water, eating more salt and fiber, and getting electrolytes from vegetables.

You Will Have Low Energy With Keto.

Many people say their concentration and energy increased after they adjusted to ketosis. Your energy might be lower at the beginning of the diet. Once your body starts producing ketones, the brain has a steady source of fuel. You should then experience better moods, increased focus, and more mental clarity.

You Should Stay on the Keto Diet Only for Short Time Periods.

When you first start a keto diet, you should stay on the diet for only two or three months, then take a break. Give your body about three weeks to adjust and then go back into the keto diet. If this works for your body, you can do this for many months or years. It all depends on how your body feels.

You Can Cheat on the Keto Diet.

It is unrealistic to stick with the keto diet all the time. Other diets encourage cheat days to give you a break or support your metabolism. However, cheating while on the keto diet might take you out of ketosis.

This might not be a problem if you do it intentionally. If you are aware that it is happening and you adjust your diet, coming out of the keto diet is fine every now and then. If you realize that you aren't in ketosis because you have been cheating and eating more carbs, just take a few days to get back into eating more fats and cutting back on the carbs.

You Can Eat Any Fat on Keto, Like You Do with Atkins.

Though, with keto, most of your calories come from fat, you can't consume all the saturated fats you want. Because keto isn't just about losing weight, you can eat healthy fats. Atkins allows any fatty foods. Many people who follow the keto diet like to stay away from processed meats such as sausage, salami, and bacon.

If you want to get more out of this diet, you can eat clean and stay away from cheeses, poor quality meats, fried food, fast food, processed food, and trans fats. To eat healthily, choose organic, cage-free eggs, wild-caught fish, pasture-raised poultry, nuts, avocados, grass-fed meats, grass-fed butter, and cold-pressed oils such as coconut oil or extra virgin olive oil.

Women and Men Are the Same on Keto.

Women are generally more sensitive to weight loss and dietary changes than men are. It is possible for women to follow the keto diet and be safe. They can also do intermittent fasting if they like. Women must make sure that they eat more non-starchy vegetables to replenish their nutrients and electrolytes.

Women must also reduce the number of stressors in their lives and listen to their bodies. Stress can create hormonal changes that prevent women from quickly entering ketosis. Pay attention to what your body tells you when you exercise. Exercise can affect your moods, the quality of your sleep, your energy, the amount of caffeine and alcohol you consume, the amount of time you stay in the sun, and the amount of environmental toxins to which you are exposed. If you begin feeling run down and overwhelmed, adjust your diet accordingly. If you push yourself too hard, the result might backfire on you.

You Must Fast on Keto.

Fasting isn't a requirement. If you want to follow the keto diet, you can choose whether to fast. You definitely shouldn't fast on the keto diet until your body has adjusted to ketosis. Once your body is used to eating fewer carbs, intermittent fasting could have many benefits. It can help with cravings, control hunger, detoxify your body, and speed up weight loss.

Some people think that fasting is hard to do because you will feel hungry. However, this isn't true. If you are eating the correct amounts of vegetables, protein, and fats that help you feel fuller longer, fasting will not be as challenging as people make it out to be.

You Can't Consume Alcohol While on the Keto Diet.

Wine, beer, and cocktails are loaded with carbohydrates. However, you do have options if you want to drink alcohol on the keto diet. Many dry wines, light beers, and liquors are very low in carbs.

Alcohol isn't totally out. You just have to be more conscious about what you choose. You also have to be careful when you drink because your body doesn't contain all those carbs that suck up alcohol. Therefore, you might not be as tolerant of alcohol. If you must drink, do so while eating a meal because the protein and fat will help your body absorb the alcohol and prevent a surge in blood sugar.

It's Dangerous.

As with any diet or life change, the keto diet does have downsides, but it isn't very dangerous.

Some potential problems include an increased risk of heart disease, increased cholesterol, gastrointestinal distress, decreased bone density, mineral and vitamin deficiencies, and kidney stones. You can mitigate most of these by adding supplements to your diet.

Stay hydrated and, if you want to fast, slowly ease into it. Know what your daily macros are and make sure you are hitting them. If you can do all this, you should avoid these problems.

Final Thoughts

In spite of everything you have heard about the keto diet, it is relatively safe for many people to follow long-term. If you incorporate a workout routine, it can help you build muscle. You could have increased energy due to the fact that the body is burning more fats.

Many people think that you can only lose weight on the keto diet. The keto diet causes very low energy and a multitude of other problems. It is thought to be unsafe for women to follow for a long time because it can lead to loss of muscles.

The keto diet is very low in carbs and very high in fats, which changes the way the body burns fat for energy. It goes from burning the sugar and carbs we consume to burning the fat we store in the body.

Everything You Need to Know

Most of these questions have been answered throughout this book. However, this section is a quick reference to the most common questions people have about the keto diet. If you want more in-depth answers, find the chapter about your question.

- How Soon Will I Be In Ketosis?

You can't simply pick and choose when you will follow the keto diet. Your body must adjust to the diet before it gets into ketosis, and this will take time – anywhere from two to seven days. It all depends on what you eat, your activity level, and your body type. The quickest way to get your body into ketosis is to exercise before you eat anything. Restrict your carb intake to less than 20 grams per day. Remember to drink plenty of water.

- Where Can I Find Recipes for a Keto Diet?

You will find a few recipes in this book. Almost any health-conscious website will have recipes, too. Just Google what you are craving, and you will be amazed at the number of recipes that pop up. You can convert your favorite recipes into low-carb versions simply by getting rid of the sugar and fruit they contain. Substitute artificial sweetener for sugar, and omit the fruit.

- How Do I Track My Intake of Carbs?

The easiest way to track your intake of carbs is by using MyFitnessPal along with its mobile app. The app doesn't let you track net carbs, but you can track the total carbs you eat along with your total fiber. You can calculate net carbs by subtracting fiber intake from total carb intake. Other apps, like FatSecret, will track your carb intake. Just research and find one that fits your lifestyle.

- Should I Count Calories?

Yes, calories matter. The number of calories you take in and work off might seem to be an easy equation, but this isn't true for everybody. Food sensitivities, endocrine disorders, and metabolic disorders all play a role in this. So, what should you do? Eat right. Never get into a deficit with calories and don't eat foods on the bad list.

On a keto diet, you usually don't have to worry about calories because proteins and fats fill you up and keep you full longer. If you like to exercise, make sure your calories don't go into a deficit. Eat enough to make up for what you lost when you exercised.

- Am I Eating Too Much Fat?

Yes, it is possible to eat too much fat. To lose weight, you must be in a deficit for calories. Eating too much fat will push you over the deficit and make you go into surplus, which causes you to gain weight. Many people can't overeat on the keto diet because it is low in carbs but high in fats.

Find a keto calculator to help you calculate your macros. This way, you can see how many carbs, proteins, and fats you must consume each day. Remember that when you do this, you can change the amount of carbs and proteins you need according to your activity level.

- Will I Lose a Lot of Weight?

The amount of weight you lose is up to you. As stated earlier, exercising will cause you to lose more weight. You can cut out foods that will cause your weight loss to stall, like dairy, artificial sweeteners, and wheat products. Wheat products include anything with identifiable wheat product, wheat flours, and wheat gluten.

Water weight loss is normal when you begin a keto diet. Ketosis has a diuretic effect on the body that can help you lose a significant amount of weight in just a few days. Remember, you are not losing fat at this point, only water. This shows that your body is beginning to turn itself into a fat burning machine.

- How Will I Know if I Am in Ketosis?

Most people use Ketostix to help them determine whether they are in ketosis. You can find these in most pharmacies. However, they are very inaccurate. Ketostix can generally let you know whether you are in ketosis. Purple and pink results on the stick show that your body is producing ketones. If the color is darker, you are probably dehydrated, and your ketone levels are very concentrated.

The Ketostix measure the amount of acetone in your urine. These are also un-used ketones. The ketone that your brain and body use for energy is called BHB or Beta-hydroxybutyrate. Ketostix do not measure this.

If you want more accurate and reliable results, use a blood ketone meter. This shows the correct amount of ketones in your blood. Hydration doesn't change them.

For more in-depth information, refer back to the chapter about ketosis.

- How Does Ketosis Work?

Ketosis happens when we don't consume carbohydrates. When we don't eat carbs, our bodies begin consuming our stored body fat for their energy needs. It's extremely healthy for us, plus it's better for the brain.

How can we get energy from fats? When we get into ketosis, our livers break down fats into ketones. These ketones give us the energy we need.

So, how does all this equal weight loss? With a calorie deficit, we are not giving our bodies the energy they need. Therefore, the body has to dig into stored fats to produce the energy we need.

- Could I Have a Heart Attack from Eating Too Much Fat?

The three groups of fats we will be consuming are monounsaturated fats, polyunsaturated fats, and saturated fats. It was once believed that saturated fats were bad for us because of the link between them and heart disease. In more re-cent years, studies have shown that saturated fats do NOT cause heart attacks but actually improve cholesterol levels. You can consume saturated fats without any worries.

Polyunsaturated fats can be a little trickier. Processed polyunsaturated fats such as vegetable oils and margarine spreads are horrible for us. They usually contain trans fats and actually have a connection to heart disease. We must avoid them at all costs. Some polyunsaturated fats occur naturally in foods like fish, which can improve cholesterol. You must find as many of these healthy fats as possible and stop eating the unhealthy ones.

Monounsaturated fats are known as the healthy ones. Olive oil is the primary example of an oil that is more of a monounsaturated fat than anything else. It is extremely healthy and can help lower cholesterol.

- Macros: Do I Need to Count Them?

"Macros" stands for "macronutrients." The main macronutrients are carbohydrates, proteins, and fats. As stated earlier, calories matter, and you must track them when you begin this lifestyle. This will not only get you into the habit of watching them, but let you see how well you are doing. It's amazing how much we lie to ourselves about the large number of carbs that sneak into our diet.

Keeping track of your macros can help if your weight loss stalls. You can easily see the things in your diet that might be causing this problem. When tracking macros, use grams and not percentages. Many newbies think that because their diet consisted of 75 percent fat, 20 percent protein, and five percent carbs, they did well. This isn't true. Grams will give you a more accurate description of what you ate.

If you get off some of your macros, it isn't a big deal. Most of the time, you have some wiggle room to go down or up by 10 to 15 grams of proteins or fats. If you sometimes go over or under, don't worry. If you are keeping your calories under control, and they aren't in the deficit too much, you will be fine.

- I'm Feeling Crappy. What Should I Do?

Often, people just starting on the keto diet experience brain fogginess and headaches. Because ketosis makes us urinate a lot, we lose a lot of water. Add the fact that our bodies are burning up fat stores, and you have the potential for disaster. You are urinating a lot of electrolytes, and you must replace them.

Eat more salt and stay hydrated. Salty foods such as salted nuts, deli meat, and bacon, along with broth, are good to drink and eat while your body is transitioning to ketosis. These will keep you functional and sane.

- What Should I Do About Constipation?

It's normal for people starting the keto diet to have irregular bowel movements. Here's a list of advice to help with constipation or bowel problems.

- Drink tea or coffee.
- Eat flax or chia seeds.
- Eat more high-fiber vegetables.
- Quit eating nuts (if you've been eating a lot).
- Consume one tablespoon of coconut oil.
- Drink more water.
- Try a magnesium supplement.

- What About Alcohol?

You can drink alcohol while on a keto diet, but be careful. Certain types of alcohol contain carbs.

If you must drink, go for liquor. Stay away from cocktails, beer, and wine, as these all contain carbs. Clear liquor is best, but stay away from flavored liquors. Those might have carbs as well.

- My Weight Loss Has Stalled. What Should I Do?

Everybody who has ever dieted has reached a weight loss plateau. Several things might have caused this problem. You can do many things to get out of this plateau, such as fat fasting, intermittent fasting, changing your eating habits, and cutting out certain foods.

Here are some suggestions that can help you lose weight again:

- Change to measuring and not weighing.
- Cut out processed foods.
- Check all foods for hidden carbs.
- Stop eating artificial sweeteners.
- Don't eat nuts.

- Lower the number of carbs you are consuming.
- Increase your fat intake.
- Stop consuming dairy.

- Do I Need to Worry if I Exercise?

Generally, two types of people exercise: people who lift weights and people who run. If you do a lot of cardio, like running marathons, biking, or running, you don't have to worry. The keto diet does not affect endurance training.

If you lift weights, you must know your end goal. Carbs can help your performance and promote muscle recovery. This means you get better strength performance and faster gains during your sessions. You can do this one of two ways: CKD and TKD.

CKD is the cyclical ketogenic diet. It is a more advanced technique. If you are new to keto, you should not do this. This is more for competitors and bodybuilders who want to do keto while building muscle during workouts. For this method, you follow a normal keto diet for five days, then change to eating more carbs for two days. You will be replenishing all the glycogen stores in your body to help you with the training you will be doing the other five days. Your goal is to get rid of all the stored glycogen.

TKD is the targeted ketogenic diet. This is where you eat carbs right before you work out, to stop ketosis while you are exercising. This works by giving your muscles a supply of glycogen to use during the workout. When you have used up all the glycogen, you will go back into ketosis.

- Do I Need to Take Supplements?

Once you've started a ketogenic diet, you might feel crampy or not like your normal self. Here are some supplements that can help you:

- Potassium Supplement
- Vitamin D Supplement
- Vitamin B Complex

- Magnesium Supplement
- Multivitamin for Men
- Multivitamin for Women

Talk with your doctor before you add supplements or vitamins to your diet.

What to Eat on Keto

You have all the information you need about what a keto diet is, so now let's look at exactly what you can and can't eat while on a keto diet.

What to Eat

- Meats – All unprocessed meats are low in carbs and great for keto. The best are grass-fed and organic meats. You're supposed to eat foods that are high in fats and not proteins, so don't go crazy. Watch out for processed meats like meatballs, sausages, and cold cuts, which sometimes have added carbs.
- Seafood and fish – These are great options, especially salmon, which is high in fat.
- Eggs – These are great because you can fix them in a variety of ways.
- High-fat sauces – A lot of the fat you consume should come from natural sources like eggs, fish, and meat. However, you can also use fats – such as coconut oil and butter – to cook.
- Above-ground vegetables – Choose vegetables that are grown above the ground, especially green vegetables. The best are:
    - Cauliflower
    - Cabbage
    - Avocado
    - Broccoli
    - Zucchini
    - Spinach
    - Asparagus
    - Kale
    - Green beans
    - Brussels sprouts

- High-fat dairy – The more fat, the better. Butter is the best, and high-fat cheeses are good, too. Consume high-fat yogurts in moderation.

Regular milk has too much sugar, so avoid it.

- Nuts – You can have these in moderation. The best are macadamia nuts, Brazil nuts, and pecans.
- Berries – These are good in moderation. They include raspberries, blackberries, strawberries, and blueberries.
- Water – This is a must-have.
- Coffee – Don't add anything except for butter or coconut oil.
- Tea – Consume any tea you like; just don't add sugar.
- Bone broth – This can add electrolytes and nutrients.
- Alcohol – If you must have alcohol, try dry wine, vodka, brandy, whiskey, and anything that doesn't have added sugar.
- Dark chocolate – Aim for chocolate that has a cocoa amount of over 70 percent. Eighty-five percent is the ideal cocoa amount.

Foods to Avoid

- Sugar – This is the biggest no-no. You must get rid of vitamin water, sports drinks, fruit juices, and soft drinks. Also:
  - Breakfast cereals
  - Frozen treats
  - Donuts
  - Chocolate bars
  - Cookies
  - Cakes
  - Candy
  - Sweets

- Starch:
  - Muesli
  - Porridge
  - Potato chips
  - French fries
  - Sweet potatoes
  - Potatoes

- Rice
- Pasta
- Bread
- Lentils
- Beans

- Beer – This is basically liquid bread.

- Fruits
- Margarine – Use real butter, not fake butter.
- Pre-packaged low-carb foods – Read the label before you buy these. Even Atkins products aren't all low-carb.

Keto Shopping List

To help you start your diet, this chapter provides a shopping list of everything you'll need. The list is organized by types of food to help make your travels through the grocery store easier.

- Meats
    - Pepperoni
    - Luncheon meats – Read the label to see if they have added nitrites or carbs
    - Hot dogs
    - Bratwurst
    - Elk
    - Buffalo
    - Venison
    - Ground lamb
    - Lamb chops
    - Pork steaks
    - Ham steaks
    - Ground pork
    - Pork ribs
    - Polish sausage
    - Kielbasa
    - Bacon
    - Breakfast sausage
    - Duck
    - Whole chicken
    - Chicken breast
    - Chicken thighs
    - Ribeye steak
    - Chuck roast
    - Ground beef 80/20

- Seafood
  - Trout
  - Tuna
  - Shrimp
  - Salmon

- Vegetables

- Zucchini
- Summer squash
- Spaghetti squash
- Sprouts
- Garlic
- Onions
- Lettuce
- Cucumbers
- Bell pepper
- Cabbage
- Cauliflower
- Broccoli

- Fruits

- Strawberries
- Raspberries
- Blackberries
- Blueberries
- Avocados

- Fats and oils
  - Sesame oil
  - Coconut oil
  - Grapeseed oil
  - Olive oil
  - Avocado oil

- Dairy
    - Greek yogurt
    - Hard cheeses
    - Butter
    - Sour cream
    - Eggs
    - Cream cheese
    - Heavy cream

- Miscellaneous

- Pork rinds
- Olives
- Beef jerky
- Full-fat ranch dressing
- Sugar-free salad dressing
- Salsa
- Hot sauce
- Cider vinegar
- Mustard
- Pickle juice
- Sugar-free pickles
- Chicken stock
- No-sugar-added sauces
- Nut flours
- Seeds
- Nuts
- Almond butter
- Sunflower butter
- Peanut butter

14-Day Plan

TO HELP YOU START YOUR keto journey, this chapter gives you a two-week plan. You will get 42 recipes, all of which state the macros as well as the serving size. If a recipe does not state a serving size, it creates a single serving. If you want to avoid having to cook as often, you can do a couple of things:

- Make lunch easy by cooking two servings of dinner the night before. Refrigerate the second serving and have it for lunch the next day.
- Make breakfast easier by choosing one keto breakfast that you really like and eating it every day. Another option is to simply drink coffee and skip breakfast if you aren't hungry.

Drink plenty of water and add plenty of salt to replenish the electrolytes you won't be getting from food.

Day One:

- Breakfast – Scrambled Eggs
- Lunch – Asian Beef Salad
- Dinner – Pesto Chicken Casserole

Day Two:

- Breakfast – Cheese Roll-Ups
- Lunch – Caprese Omelet
- Dinner – Meat Pie

Day Three:

- Breakfast – Frittata
- Lunch – Chicken Soup

- Dinner – Carbonara

Day Four:

- Breakfast – Keto Latte
- Lunch – Avocado Salad
- Dinner – Pizza

Day Five:

- Breakfast – Mushroom Omelet
- Lunch – Smoked Salmon Plate
- Dinner – Keto Tacos

Day Six:

- Breakfast – Baked Bacon Omelet
- Lunch – Quesadillas
- Dinner – Asian Cabbage Stir-Fry

Day Seven:

- Breakfast – Pancakes
- Lunch – Italian Plate
- Dinner – Pork Chops

Day Eight:

- Breakfast – Breakfast Sandwich
- Lunch – Tuna Salad
- Dinner – Hamburger with Tomato Sauce

Day Nine:

- Breakfast – Bulletproof Coffee
- Lunch – Roast Beef

- Dinner – Fried Salmon

Day Ten:

- Breakfast – Coconut Porridge
- Lunch – Shrimp and Artichoke
- Dinner – Chicken Casserole

Day Eleven:

- Breakfast – Egg Muffins
- Lunch – Cauliflower Soup
- Dinner - Cheeseburger

Day Twelve:

- Breakfast – Boiled Eggs
- Lunch – Caesar Salad
- Dinner – Fat Head Pizza

Day Thirteen:

- Breakfast – Bacon and Eggs
- Lunch – Salmon-Filled Avocado
- Dinner – Ribeye Steak and Veggies

Day Fourteen:

- Breakfast – Western Omelet
- Lunch – Prosciutto-Wrapped Asparagus
- Dinner – Creamy Fish Casserole

Meals

Asian Beef Salad

WHAT YOU WILL NEED:

- Ribeye steaks, ⅔ pound
- Chili flakes, 1 teaspoon
- Grated ginger, 1 tablespoon
- Fish sauce, 1 tablespoon
- Olive oil, 1 tablespoon

Salad:

- Sesame seeds, 1 tablespoon
- Cilantro
- Red onion, half
- Lettuce, 3 ounces
- Cucumber, 2 ounces
- Cherry tomatoes, 3 ounces
- Scallions, 2

Mayo:

- Pepper
- Salt
- Lime juice, ½ tablespoon
- Sesame oil, 1 tablespoon
- Olive oil, ½ cup
- Dijon mustard, 1 teaspoon
- Egg yolk

What you will do:

1. Mix the mustard and egg yolk together. As you whisk, slowly add

the olive oil. This can be done either with an immersion blender or by hand. Once the mayo has become emulsified, add the sesame oil, spices, and lime juice. Set the mayo to the side.

2. Mix together the olive oil, chili flakes, ginger, and fish sauce and add it to a plastic bag. Add the rib eye and let it marinate for 15 minutes.

3. Chop up all the ingredients for the salad, minus the scallions. Split them between 2 plates.

4. Heat a skillet and add the sesame seeds. Allow them to dry roast for a few minutes. Place them to the side.

5. Pat off the meat and fry in the skillet for a few minutes on each side. Cook to your desired doneness (though this dish is best cooked to medium).

6. Fry the scallions for a bit in the skillet.

7. Cut the steak into thin slices. Add the scallions and beef to the top of the vegetables and top with the sesame seeds. Serve with the mayo.

> **7 grams – net carb**

> **98 grams – fat**

> **34 grams – protein**

> **2 servings**

Pesto Chicken Casserole

What you will need:

- Pepper
- Salt
- Chopped garlic clove
- Diced feta, 8 ounces
- Pitted olives, ½ cup
- Heavy whipping cream, 1½ cups
- Pesto, 3 ounces
- Butter, 2 ounces
- Chicken, 25 ounces
- Olive oil, 4 tablespoons
- Leafy greens, 5.33 ounces

What you will do:

1. Set your oven to 400. Slice the chicken into cubes and season with pepper and salt.

1. Place the butter in a skillet and fry the chicken in batches until browned. Combine the heavy cream and pesto in a bowl.
2. Add the chicken cubes in a casserole dish along with the garlic, feta, and olives. Drizzle everything with the pesto mixture.
3. Let this bake for 20 to 30 minutes, or until bubbly and browned along the edges.

› **7 grams – net carb**

› **110 grams – fat**

› **42 grams - protein**

› **4 servings**

Caprese Omelet

What you will need:

- Olive oil, 2 tablespoons
- Mozzarella cheese, 5 ounces
- Halved cherry tomatoes, 3 ounces
- Basil, 1 tablespoon
- Pepper
- Salt
- Eggs, 6

What you will do:

1. Break the eggs into a bowl, add pepper and salt, and whisk together. Stir in the basil. Make sure the tomatoes are halved and the cheese is diced.

1. Heat a skillet with the oil and fry the tomatoes for a bit. Remove the tomatoes. Add the eggs to the skillet and top with the tomatoes. Allow to cook until the eggs firm up a bit. Top with the cheese.
2. Turn the heat down and allow it to cook until the egg is completely set. Remove from the pan and serve.

> **4 grams – net carb**

> **43 grams – fat**

> **33 grams – protein**

> **2 servings**

Meat Pie

What you will need:

- Water, ½ cup
- Tomato paste, 4 tablespoons
- Dried oregano, 1 tablespoon
- Pepper
- Salt
- Ground beef, 20 ounces
- Butter, 2 tablespoons
- Chopped garlic clove
- Chopped onion, half

Crust:

- Water, 4 tablespoons
- Egg
- Olive oil, 3 tablespoons
- Pinch salt
- Baking powder, 1 teaspoon
- Ground psyllium husk powder, 1 tablespoon
- Coconut flour, 4 tablespoons
- Sesame seeds, 4 tablespoons
- Almond flour, ¾ cup

Topping:

- Shredded cheese, 7 ounces
- Cottage cheese, 8 ounces

What you will do:

1. Set your oven to 350. Add the butter to a skillet and cook the garlic and onion until the onion becomes soft. Add the beef and cook until

browned. Mix in the pepper, oregano, basil, and salt.

1. Mix in the tomato paste and water. Turn down the heat and let it simmer for 20 minutes. As this is cooking, make the crust.
2. Place all the dough ingredients in a food processor and combine until it forms a ball. You can do this by hand if you don't have a processor.
3. Grease a springform pan and lay a piece of parchment paper in the bottom. Spread the dough onto the bottom and the sides with greased fingers. Let this bake for 10 to 15 minutes. Pour the meat mixture into the baked crust.
4. Mix the topping ingredients and spread them across the meat. Allow the pie to bake for 30 to 40 minutes, or until it becomes golden.

> **7 grams – net carb**

> **47 grams – fat**

> **38 grams – protein**

> **6 servings**

Chicken Soup

What you will need:

- Sliced green cabbage, 2 cups
- Shredded chickens, 2 cups
- Medium carrot
- Chicken broth, 8 cups
- Pepper, ¼ teaspoon
- Salt, 1 teaspoon
- Dried parsley, 2 teaspoons
- Dried minced onion, 2 tablespoons
- Minced garlic cloves, 2
- Sliced mushrooms, 6 ounces
- Celery stalks, 2
- Butter, 4 ounces

What you will do:

1. Add the butter to a pot and melt. Slice the mushrooms and celery. Add the garlic, mushrooms, celery, and dried onion to the pot and let them cook for 3 to 4 minutes.

1. Add the pepper, broth, salt, parsley, and carrot. Let this simmer until the veggies become tender.
2. Add the cabbage and chicken and let it simmer for another 8 to 12 minutes, or until the cabbage is tender.

> **4 grams – net carb**

> **40 grams – fat**

> **33 grams – protein**

> **8 servings**

Carbonara

What you will need:

- Grated parmesan, 3 ounces
- Egg yolks, 4
- Zucchini, 30 ounces
- Chopped parsley
- Pepper
- Salt
- Mayonnaise, ¼ cup
- Heavy whipping cream, 1¼ cup
- Butter, 1 tablespoon
- Diced bacon, 10 ounces

What you will do:

1. Add the cream to a pot and let it come to a boil. Turn down the heat and boil for a couple of minutes until it has reduced by a fourth.

1. Cook the bacon until crispy, reserving the fat for later use.
2. Combine the mayo with the cream and add pepper and salt. Let this cook until the mayonnaise has warmed. Use a spiralizer to turn the zucchini into noodles. You can also create strips with a potato peeler.
3. Place the noodles in the cream sauce. Divide this between 4 bowls and top each with parsley, egg yolk, bacon, and parmesan.
4. Drizzle the tops with bacon grease, and enjoy.

> **9 grams – net carb**

> **80 grams – fat**

> **25 grams – protein**

> **4 servings**

Avocado Salad

WHAT YOU WILL NEED:

- Arugula, 4 ounces
- Walnuts, 4 ounces
- Avocados, 2
- Bacon, 8 ounces
- Goat cheese, 8 ounces
- Dressing:
- Heavy whipping cream, 2 tablespoons
- Olive oil, ½ cup
- Mayonnaise, ½ cup
- Juice of half lemon

What you will do:

1. Set your oven to 400 and line a baking dish with parchment paper. Slice the goat cheese into ½-inch slices and lay in the baking dish. Let this bake until golden.

1. Cook the bacon until crispy.
2. Divide the arugula among four plates and top with sliced avocado. Top with the goat cheese and bacon. Sprinkle with the walnuts.
3. Add all the dressing ingredients to a blender and mix until combined. Add pepper and salt to taste. Serve the salads with a drizzle of dressing.

> 6 grams – net carb

> 123 grams – fat

> 27 grams – protein

> 4 servings

Pizza

What you will need:

- Olives
- Pepperoni, 1½ ounces
- Shredded cheese, 5 ounces
- Oregano, 1 teaspoon
- Tomato paste, 3 tablespoons
- Shredded cheese, 6 ounces
- Eggs, 4

What you will do:

1. Set your oven to 400. Crack the eggs into a bowl and stir in the 6 ounces of shredded cheese. Make sure they are well-combined.

1. Line a baking sheet with parchment paper and spread the cheese batter into a thin crust. You can also make two round crusts if you want. Let this bake for 15 minutes. Remove and let the crust cool for a bit.
2. Increase the temperature of the oven to 450.
3. Top the crust with the tomato paste. Sprinkle on the oregano. Top with the remaining cheese, pepperoni, and olives.
4. Let this bake for 5 to 10 minutes. Serve with a fresh salad.

> **8 grams – net carb**

> **90 grams – fat**

> **55 grams – protein**

> **2 servings**

Smoked Salmon Plate

What you will need:

- Pepper
- Salt
- Lime, half
- Olive oil, 1 tablespoon
- Baby spinach, 2 ounces
- Mayonnaise, 1 cup
- Smoked salmon, ¾ pound

What you will do:

1. Separate the spinach and salmon on 2 plates. Serve with a dollop of mayo and a wedge of lime.
2. Drizzle the spinach with olive oil and season with pepper and salt.

> **1 gram – net carb**

> **109 grams – fat**

> **105 grams – protein**

> **2 servings**

Keto Tacos

What you will need:

Beef:

- Pepper
- Salt
- Water, 1 cup
- Taco seasoning, 2 tablespoons
- Olive oil, 2 tablespoons
- Ground beef, 1 pound

Salsa:

- Pepper
- Salt
- Juice of 1 lime
- Olive oil, 1 tablespoon
- Chopped cilantro, ½ cup
- Diced tomato
- Avocados, 2

Tortillas:

- Salt, ½ teaspoon
- Coconut flour, 1 tablespoon
- Ground psyllium husk powder, 1½ teaspoons
- Cream cheese, 5 ounces
- Egg whites, 2
- Eggs, 2

Serving:

- Shredded lettuce, 3 ounces
- Shredded cheese, 1½ cups

===========

WHAT YOU WILL DO:

1. Set your oven to 400. Beat the egg whites and eggs together, mixing for a few minutes. Add the cream cheese and mix until smooth. Add the coconut flour, psyllium husk, and salt. Add the coconut flour a spoonful at a time. Allow this to sit for a few minutes. It should thicken to a pancake batter consistency.

1. Line 2 baking sheets with parchment. Spread the batter into ¼-inch thick circles. It should make 4 to 6 circles. Let this bake for 5 minutes, or until it's browned on the edges. Make sure they don't burn.
2. Heat the oil in a skillet and cook the beef until browned. Mix in the water and taco seasoning. Allow this to simmer until the water evaporates.
3. Dice the salsa ingredients and mix them together. Season with cilantro, pepper, salt, olive oil, and lime juice.
4. Top your tortillas with the meat, salsa, cheese, and lettuce.

> **9 grams – net carb**

> **66 grams – fat**

> **42 grams – protein**

> **4 servings**

Quesadillas

What you will need:

- Olive oil, 1 tablespoon
- Leafy greens, 1 ounce
- Grated Mexican cheese, 5 ounces
- Keto tortillas, 6

What you will do:

1. Find the recipe for the keto tortillas in the keto tacos recipe above.

1. Add the oil to a skillet and add a tortilla. Sprinkle it with some cheese and add some leafy greens. Top with more cheese and another tortilla. Fry for a minute on both sides. Enjoy.

> **5 grams – net carb**

> **41 grams – fat**

> **21 grams – protein**

> **3 servings**

Asian Cabbage Stir-Fry

What you will need:

- Sesame oil, 1 tablespoon
- Grated ginger, 1 tablespoon
- Chili flakes, 1 teaspoon
- Sliced scallions, 3
- Garlic cloves, 2
- White wine vinegar, 1 tablespoon
- Pepper, ¼ teaspoon
- Onion powder, 1 teaspoon
- Salt, 1 teaspoon
- Ground beef, 20 ounces
- Butter, 5 ounces
- Green cabbage, 25 ounces
- Wasabi paste, ½ tablespoon
- Mayonnaise, 1 cup

What you will do:

1. Finely shred the cabbage. Fry the cabbage in a couple of ounces of butter. Make sure it doesn't brown up. It should just soften. Add the vinegar and spices. Stir fry for a few more minutes. Place the cabbage in a bowl. Add the remaining butter to the pan and mix in the ginger, chili flakes, and garlic. Let them sauté for a few minutes.

1. Mix in the beef and cook thoroughly. Turn down the heat and add the cabbage and scallions. Mix everything and season with pepper and salt. Drizzle with some sesame oil. Combine the mayo and wasabi. Serve the stir-fry topped with mayonnaise.

> **9 grams – net carb**

> **93 grams – fat**

> 33 grams – protein

> 4 servings

Italian Plate

What you will need:

- Pepper
- Salt
- Green olive, 10
- Olive oil, ⅓ cup
- Tomatoes, 2
- Prosciutto, 7 ounces
- Mozzarella cheese, 7 ounces

What you will do:

1. Divide the ingredients between 2 plates and drizzle with olive oil.
2. Sprinkle with pepper and salt. Enjoy.

> **8 grams – net carb**

> **69 grams – fat**

> **40 grams – protein**

> **2 servings**

Pork Chops

What you will need:

- Pepper
- Salt
- Green beans, 1 pound
- Butter, 2 ounces
- Pork chops, 4

Garlic butter:

- Pepper
- Salt
- Lemon juice, 1 tablespoon
- Garlic powder, ½ tablespoon
- Dried parsley, 1 tablespoon
- Butter, 5 ounces

What you will do:

1. Let the butter for the garlic butter come to room temperature.

1. Combine the lemon juice, parsley, garlic, and butter. Season with pepper and salt and set this to the side.
2. Season your pork chops with pepper and salt. Heat a skillet and add butter. Fry the chops for around 5 minutes on both sides, or until cooked through. Take out the chops and keep warm.
3. In the same skillet, add the beans. Add pepper and salt. Cook until vibrant in color and slightly soft. Serve the chops and beans with some of the garlic butter.

> **6 grams – net carb**

> **73 grams – fat**

> **54 grams – protein**

> **4 servings**

Tuna Salad

What you will need:

- Pepper
- Salt
- Olive oil, 2 tablespoons
- Cherry tomatoes, 4 ounces
- Romaine lettuce, ½ pound
- Eggs, 4
- Dijon mustard, 1 teaspoon
- Zest and juice from half a lemon
- Mayonnaise, ¾ cup
- Tuna, 5 ounces
- Scallions, 2
- Celery stalks, 4 ounces

What you will do:

1. Finely chop the scallions and celery. Combine the celery, scallions, mustard, mayonnaise, lemon, and tuna. Add pepper and salt to taste. Set aside.

1. Place the eggs in a pot and cover with water. Allow the eggs to boil for 5 to 6 minutes for soft/medium eggs or 8 to 10 minutes for hardboiled.
2. Set them in ice water and then peel. Divide into halves. Place the lettuce in 2 bowls and top with the tuna and eggs. Add the tomatoes and drizzle with oil. Sprinkle with pepper and salt.

> **6 grams – net carb**

> **91 grams – fat**

> **33 grams – protein**

> 2 servings

Hamburger in Tomato Sauce

What you will need:

Patties:

- Butter, ¼ teaspoon
- Olive oil, 1 tablespoon
- Chopped parsley, 2 ounces
- Pepper, ¼ teaspoon
- Salt, 1 teaspoon
- Crumbled feta, 3 ounces
- Egg
- Ground beef, 25 ounces

Gravy:

- Pepper
- Salt
- Tomato paste, 2 tablespoons
- Chopped parsley, 1 ounce
- Heavy whipping cream, ¾ cup

Fried Cabbage:

- Pepper
- Salt
- Butter, 4¼ ounces
- Shredded cabbage, 25 ounces

What you will do:

1. Blend all the patty ingredients. Form the mixture into 8 patties. Place the oil and butter in a skillet and cook for 10 minutes or until cooked through. Flip them a couple of times while cooking.

1. When almost done, add the whipping cream and tomato paste to the pan. Stir and allow it to simmer for a couple of minutes. Season with pepper and salt. Sprinkle everything with parsley before serving.
2. For the cabbage: Add the butter to a skillet and fry the cabbage for 15 minutes, or until wilted and browned on the edges. Season with pepper and salt.
3. Serve the patties with the cabbage.

> **10 grams – net carb**

> **78 grams – fat**

> **43 grams – protein**

> **4 servings**

Roast Beef

What you will need:

- Pepper
- Salt
- Olive oil, 2 tablespoons
- Lettuce, 2 ounces
- Dijon mustard, 1 tablespoon
- Mayonnaise, 5 cups
- Scallion
- Radishes, 6
- Avocado
- Cheddar cheese, 5 ounces
- Deli roast beef, 7 ounces

What you will do:

1. Lay the radishes, avocado, cheese, and roast beef on 2 plates. Add the mustard, onion, and mayonnaise. Serve with lettuce and drizzle with olive oil.

> **6 grams – net carb**

> **98 grams – fat**

> **38 grams – protein**

> **2 servings**

Salmon

What you will need:

- Lime
- Salmon, 1½ pounds
- Grated cheddar cheese, 5 ounces
- Pepper
- Salt
- Butter, 3½ ounces
- Broccoli, 1 pound

What you will do:

1. Set your oven to 400, preferably a broiler.

1. Slice the broccoli into florets and cook them in salted water for a few minutes. Drain and place in a greased casserole dish. Top with butter and pepper.
2. Sprinkle on the cheese and let this bake for 15 to 20 minutes. The cheese should turn golden.
3. Fry the salmon in the butter for a few minutes on both sides. Divide the broccoli and salmon into 4 servings and serve with a wedge of lime.

> **6 grams – net carb**

> **55 grams – fat**

> **46 grams – protein**

> **4 servings**

Shrimp and Artichoke

What you will need:

- 'Pepper
- Salt
- Olive oil, 4 tablespoons
- Baby spinach, 1½ ounces
- Mayonnaise, ½ cup
- Sun-dried tomatoes, 6
- Canned artichokes, 14 ounces
- Cooked shrimp, 10 ounces
- Eggs, 4

What you will do:

1. Boil the eggs to your desired doneness. Let the eggs cool in ice water for a couple of minutes, then peel them.

1. Lay the tomatoes, artichokes, shrimp, and eggs on 2 plates and serve with mayonnaise and spinach. Drizzle with olive oil and season with pepper and salt.

> **7 grams – net carb**

> **80 grams – fat**

> **36 grams – protein**

> **2 servings**

Chicken Casserole

What you will need:

- Pepper
- Salt
- Shredded cheese, 7 ounces
- Cherry tomatoes, 4 ounces
- Leek
- Cauliflower, 1 pound
- Butter, 3 tablespoons
- Chicken thighs, 30 ounces
- Juice of half a lemon
- Green pesto, 2 tablespoons
- Heavy whipping cream, 1 cup

What you will do:

1. Set your oven to 400. Combine the lemon juice, pesto, and heavy cream. Season with pepper and salt.

1. Rub the chicken with pepper and salt and fry in the butter until golden. Add the chicken to a greased casserole dish and top with the cream mixture.
2. Chop the tomatoes, leek, and cauliflower. Add this to the top of the chicken. Sprinkle with cheese and bake for 30 minutes. The chicken should be cooked through.

> **6 grams – net carb**

> **56 grams – fat**

> **36 grams – protein**

> **6 servings**

Cauliflower Soup

What you will need:

- Pecans, 3 ounces
- Paprika, 1 teaspoon
- Butter, 1 tablespoon – for frying
- Diced bacon, 7 ounces
- Pepper
- Salt
- Butter, 4 ounces
- Dijon mustard, 1 tablespoon
- Cream cheese, 7 ounces
- Cauliflower, 15 ounces
- Chicken broth, 4 cups

What you will do:

1. Slice the cauliflower into florets. Reserve a handful of cauliflower and dice it into some bites.

1. Cook the small pieces of cauliflower and the bacon in butter. Add the paprika and nuts. Set aside for serving.
2. Boil the large pieces of cauliflower in the chicken stock until soft. Mix in the butter, mustard, and cream cheese. Use an immersion blender to mix the soup until smooth. Add pepper and salt.
3. Serve the soup topped with the bacon mixture.

> **6 grams – net carb**

> **53 grams – fat**

> **10 grams – protein**

> **6 servings**

Cheeseburger

What you will need:

- Butter, 2 ounces – for frying
- Chopped oregano, 2 tablespoons
- Paprika, 2 teaspoons
- Onion powder, 2 teaspoons
- Garlic powder, 2 teaspoons
- Shredded cheese, 7 ounces
- Ground beef, 25 ounces

Salsa:

- Cilantro
- Salt
- Olive oil, 1 tablespoon
- Avocado
- Scallions, 2
- Tomatoes, 2

Toppings:

- Pickled jalapenos, ¼ cup
- Lettuce, 5 ounces
- Sliced pickles, ½ cup
- Dijon mustard, 4 tablespoons
- Cooked bacon, 5 ounces
- Mayonnaise, ¾ cup

What you will do:

1. Chop all the ingredients for the salsa and mix them together. Set to the side.

1. Combine the beef with half the cheese and all the seasonings. Form into 4 burgers and cook however you prefer. When they are almost done, top the burgers with the remaining cheese.
2. Serve the burgers with lettuce, pickle, and mustard. Top with the salsa.

> **8 grams – net carb**

> **104 grams – fat**

> **54 grams – protein**

> **4 servings**

Caesar Salad

What you will need:

- Grated parmesan, 2 ounces
- Romaine lettuce, half head
- Bacon, 5⅓ ounces
- Pepper
- Salt
- Olive oil, 1 tablespoon
- Chicken breasts, 10 ounces

Dressing:

- Pepper
- Alt
- Chopped anchovies, 2 tablespoons
- Parmesan cheese, 2 tablespoons
- Juice and zest of half a lemon
- Dijon mustard, 1 tablespoon
- Mayonnaise, ½ cup

What you will do:

1. Mix all the dressing ingredients in a blender until smooth. Refrigerate until needed.

1. Set the oven to 400. Lay the chicken in a baking dish and season with olive oil, pepper, and salt. Let the chicken bake for 20 minutes or until cooked through.
2. Cook the bacon until crispy. Shred the lettuce and divide between 2 plates. Top with the chicken and bacon. Finish with a dollop of the dressing and some grated parmesan.

> **5 grams – net carb**

> **102 grams – fat**

> **57 grams – protein**

> **2 servings**

Fat Head Pizza

What you will need:

Crust:

- Salt, ½ teaspoon
- Egg
- White wine vinegar, 1 teaspoon
- Cream cheese, 2 tablespoons
- Almond flour, ¾ cup
- Shredded mozzarella, 1½ cups

Toppings:

- Shredded mozzarella, 1½ cups
- Oregano, ½ teaspoon
- Tomato sauce, ½ cup
- Butter, 1 tablespoon
- Italian sausage, 8 ounces

What you will do:

1. Set your oven to 400.

Crust:

1. Add the cream cheese and mozzarella to a microwavable bowl and heat for a few seconds. Stir and heat for a few seconds longer. Continue this process until they have melted together. Stir in the other crust ingredients.
2. Add some oil to your hands and flatten the dough onto parchment paper. Try to make an 8-inch circle. Prick with a fork and bake for 10 to 12 minutes, or until golden.

Pizza:

1. Cook the ground sausage in butter. Spread the tomato sauce over the crust and top with the meat and cheese. Allow this to bake for 10 to 15 minutes. Sprinkle with oregano and serve with a side salad.

> **10 grams – net carb**

> **110 grams – fat**

> **67 grams – protein**

> **2 servings**

Salmon-Filled Avocados

What you will need:

- Lemon juice, 2 tablespoons
- Pepper
- Salt
- Mayonnaise, ¾ cup
- Smoked salmon, 6 ounces
- Avocados, 2

What you will do:

1. Slice the avocados in half and take out the pits. Dollop some mayonnaise in the hole of each avocado half and top with the smoked salmon.

1. Use the lemon juice to keep the avocado from turning brown and to add a bit of flavor. Sprinkle with pepper and salt.

> **6 grams – net carb**

> **71 grams – fat**

> **58 grams – protein**

> **2 servings**

Ribeye Steak with Vegetables

What you will need:

- Pepper
- Salt
- Ribeye steaks, 1½ pound
- Dried thyme, 1 tablespoon
- Olive oil, 3 tablespoons
- Cherry tomatoes, 10 ounces
- Whole garlic head
- Broccoli, 1 pound

Anchovy Butter:

- Pepper
- Salt
- Lemon juice, 1 tablespoon
- Room-temperature butter, 5 ounces
- Anchovies, 1 ounce

What you will do:

1. For the butter: Dice the anchovies and mix them into the butter along with the pepper, salt, and lemon juice. Set to the side.

1. Set your oven to 450. Separate the garlic head into cloves, but don't peel. Slice the broccoli into florets.
2. Grease a roasting dish and add the vegetables. Drizzle with olive and add pepper and salt. Stir them to coat well and let them cook for 15 minutes.
3. Add olive oil to both sides of the steaks and season with pepper and salt. Fry them in a pan. At this point, you want to sear the outsides.
4. Take the veggies out of the oven and snuggle the steak into the veggies. Turn the heat to 400 and let them cook for 10 to 15 more minutes.

This all depends on how done you want your steaks.

5. Take them out and serve them with anchovy butter.

> **11 grams – net carb**

> **66 grams – fat**

> **41 grams – protein**

> **4 servings**

Prosciutto-Wrapped Asparagus

What you will need:

- Olive oil, 2 tablespoons
- Pepper, ¼ teaspoon
- Goat cheese, 5 ounces
- Thinly sliced prosciutto, 2 ounces
- Asparagus, 12

What you will do:

1. Set your oven to 450. Clean and trim your asparagus. Create 12 slices of goat cheese and then slice those in half again. Slice the prosciutto slices in half and wrap each around 2 pieces of cheese and 1 asparagus.

1. Lay them on a baking dish and drizzle with oil and pepper. Let them cook for 15 minutes.

> **1 gram – net carb**

> **19 grams – fat**

> **11 grams – protein**

> **4 servings**

Creamy Fish Casserole

What you will need:

- Butter, 3 ounces
- Parsley, 1 tablespoon
- Pepper, ¼ teaspoon
- Salt, 1 teaspoon
- Dijon mustard, 1 tablespoon
- Heavy whipping cream, 1¼ cup
- Whitefish, 25 ounces
- Butter – for greasing
- Capers, 2 tablespoons
- Scallions, 6
- Broccoli, 15 ounces
- Olive oil, 2 tablespoons

What you will do:

1. Set your oven to 400. Cut the broccoli into florets. Fry the broccoli for 5 minutes until soft. Add pepper and salt.

1. Add the capers and chopped scallions. Cook for another couple of minutes. Place the veggies into a greased casserole dish.
2. Place the fish in with the vegetables. Combine the mustard, whipping cream, and parsley. Pour the mixture over the fish and veggies. Top with butter slices.
3. Let this bake for 20 minutes. The fish should flake easily with a fork.

> **8 grams – net carb**

> **69 grams – fat**

> **41 grams – protein**

> **4 servings**

Breakfast

Scrambled Eggs

WHAT YOU WILL NEED:

- Butter, 1 ounce
- Eggs, 2
- Pepper
- Salt

What you will do:

1. Break the eggs into a bowl and add pepper and salt. Whisk together with a fork.

1. Add the butter to a skillet and allow it to melt. Add the eggs and cook, stirring constantly for a couple of minutes until almost cooked through. Pour out into a plate. Don't worry if they still look a little wet. The eggs will continue to cook.

> **1 gram – net carb**

> **31 grams – fat**

> **11 grams – protein**

Cheese Roll-Ups

What you will need:

- Butter, 2 ounces
- Cheddar, Edam, provolone cheese slices, 8 ounces

What you will do:

1. Let the butter reach room temperature.

1. Lay out the cheese slices. Spread the butter on top of each piece of cheese and roll them up.

> **2 grams – net carb**

> **31 grams – fat**

> **13 grams – protein**

> **4 servings**

Frittata

What you will need:

- Pepper
- Salt
- Shredded cheese, 5 ounces
- Heavy whipping cream, 1 cup
- Eggs, 8
- Fresh spinach, 8 ounces
- Butter, 2 tablespoons
- Diced bacon, 5 ounces

What you will do:

1. Set your oven to 350. Add the butter to a skillet and fry the bacon until crispy. Add the spinach and let it cook until it wilts. Take this out of the pan and set to the side.

1. Beat the cream and eggs and add to a 9-by-9 greased baking dish. You can also grease 4 ramekins and cook it in individual serving size.
2. Top the eggs with the cheese, spinach, and bacon. Slide it into the oven to cook for 25 to 30 minutes. The eggs should be set and the top golden.

> **4 grams – net carb**

> **59 grams – fat**

> **27 grams – protein**

> **4 servings**

Keto Latte

What you will need:

- Pumpkin pie spice, 1 teaspoon
- Vanilla extract, splash
- Boiling water, 1½ cups
- Coconut oil, 2 tablespoons
- Eggs, 2

What you will do:

1. Place all the ingredients in a blender and mix everything together. Enjoy immediately.

> **1 gram – net carb**

> **18 grams – fat**

> **6 grams – protein**

> **2 servings**

Mushroom Omelet

What you will need:

- Pepper
- Salt
- Mushrooms, 3
- Diced onion, 3 tablespoons
- Shredded cheese, 1 ounce
- Butter, 1 ounce
- Eggs, 3

What you will do:

1. Beat the eggs together with pepper and salt. Add the butter to a skillet. Once it has melted, add the eggs.
2. Once the omelet has firmed up but is still a bit raw, add the onion, mushrooms, and cheese.
3. Once the egg is completely cooked, fold the egg in half and slide onto a plate.

> **4 grams – net carb**

> **43 grams – fat**

> **25 grams – protein**

Baked Bacon Omelet

What you will need:

- Pepper
- Salt
- Chopped chives, 1 tablespoon
- Spinach, 2 ounces
- Butter, 3 ounces
- Cubed bacon, 5 ounces
- Eggs, 4

What you will do:

1. Set your oven to 400 and grease 2 ramekins with butter. Cook the spinach and bacon in the remaining butter.
2. Beat the eggs until frothy and stir in the bacon and spinach. Make sure you also use the fat from frying.
3. Add a few chives and top with pepper and salt. Separate the batter into the ramekins and allow them to cook for 20 minutes, or until cooked through. Let cool for a bit and enjoy.

> **2 grams – net carb**

> **72 grams – fat**

> **21 grams – protein**

> **2 servings**

Pancakes

What you will need:

- Heavy whipping cream, 1 cup
- Fresh berries, ½ cup
- Butter, 2 ounces
- Ground psyllium husk powder, 1 tablespoon
- Cottage cheese, 7 ounces
- Eggs, 4

What you will do:

1. Mix the psyllium husk powder, cottage cheese, and eggs. Allow this to thicken for 5 to 10 minutes.
2. Add the butter to a skillet and fry the pancakes for 3 to 4 minutes on both sides. Keep the size small so you can flip them.
3. Beat the whipping cream until it forms soft peaks.
4. Serve your pancakes with the whipped cream and berries.

> **5 grams – net carb**

> **39 grams – fat**

> **13 grams – protein**

> **4 servings**

Breakfast Sandwich

What you will need:

- Tabasco
- Pepper
- Salt
- Cheddar cheese slices, 2 ounces
- Smoked deli ham, 1 ounce
- Eggs, 4
- Butter, 2 tablespoons

What you will do:

1. Place the butter in a skillet. Fry each of the eggs in the skillet until done to your liking. Make sure you pepper and salt them.
2. The fried eggs are the bread for your sandwich. Add the deli ham and cheese, then top with a second egg. Sprinkle with some Tabasco sauce if you want.

> **2 grams – net carb**

> **30 grams – fat**

> **20 grams – protein**

> **2 servings**

Bulletproof Coffee

What you will need:

- Coconut oil, 1 tablespoon
- Unsalted butter, 2 tablespoons
- Hot coffee, 1 cup

What you will do:

1. Blend all the ingredients in your blender until frothy and enjoy.

> **0 grams – net carb**

> **38 grams – fat**

> **1 gram – protein**

Coconut Porridge

What you will need:

- Pinch salt
- Coconut cream, 4 tablespoons
- Pinch ground psyllium husk powder
- Coconut flour, 1 tablespoon
- Egg
- Butter, 1 ounce

What you will do:

1. Place all the ingredients in a pot. Mix everything and let it heat over low. Stir constantly until it reaches your desired texture. Serve with coconut milk and berries if you want.

> **4 grams – net carb**

> **49 grams – fat**

> **9 grams – protein**

Egg Muffins

What you will need:

- Pepper
- Salt
- Pesto, 2 tablespoons
- Shredded cheese, 6 ounces
- Cooked bacon, 5 ounces
- Chipped scallions, 2
- Eggs, 12

What you will do:

1. Set your oven to 350. Grease a muffin tin with butter. Chop the scallions and bacon and place them in the bottom of the tin.
2. Beat the pesto, seasonings, and eggs. Add the cheese and mix well. Pour this into the muffin tin over the bacon. Let it cook for 15 to 20 minutes. Cool slightly. Carefully remove the muffins.

> **2 grams – net carb**

> **26 grams – fat**

> **23 grams – protein**

> **6 servings**

Boiled Eggs

What you will need:

- Avocado – optional
- Mayonnaise, 8 tablespoons
- Eggs, 8

What you will do:

1. Place the eggs in water and bring to a boil. Allow them to cook to your desired doneness: 10 minutes for hard-boiled, 8 minutes for medium, and 6 minutes for soft-boiled.
2. Each person gets 2 eggs with 2 tablespoons of mayonnaise. Serve with avocado if desired.

> **1 gram – net carb**

> **29 grams – fat**

> **11 grams – protein**

> **4 servings**

Bacon and Eggs

What you will need:

- Sliced bacon, 5 ounces
- Eggs, 8

What you will do:

1. Fry the bacon until crispy. Set to the side. Leave the fat it created in the skillet.
2. In the same pan, fry the eggs. Cook them however you'd like: scrambled, sunny side up, over easy, etc. Season with pepper and salt and enjoy.

> **1 gram – net carb**

> **22 grams – fat**

> **15 grams – protein**

> **4 servings**

Western Omelet

What you will need:

- Diced deli ham, 5 ounces
- Chopped bell pepper, half
- Chopped onion, half
- Butter, 2 ounces
- Shredded cheese, 3 ounces
- Pepper
- Salt
- Heavy whipping cream, 2 tablespoons
- Eggs, 6

What you will do:

1. Beat the eggs, heavy cream, pepper, and salt until frothy. Mix in half of the shredded cheese.
2. Add the butter to a skillet and cook the ham, peppers, and onion. Pour in the egg mixture and cook until almost firm.
3. Turn down the heat and top with the remaining cheese. Fold in half and enjoy.

> **6 grams – net carb**

> **58 grams – fat**

> **40 grams – protein**

> **2 servings**

Desserts and Snacks

Parmesan Chips

WHAT YOU WILL NEED:

- Pumpkin seeds, 2/3 ounce
- Flaxseeds, 2/3 ounce
- Chia seeds, 2/3 ounce
- Grated parmesan, 2/3 cup

What you will do:

1. Set your oven to 350. Add parchment paper to a baking sheet. Combine all the ingredients.
2. Place small mounds of the mixture on the baking sheet. Leave space between them and do not flatten the mounds. Allow them to bake for 10 to 15 minutes. Check on them often. Take them out once they brown slightly.
3. Let them cool before removing them from the paper.

> **3 grams – net carb**

> **25 grams – fat**

> **24 grams – protein**

> **2 servings**

Avocado Hummus

What you will need:

- Pepper, ¼ teaspoon
- Salt, ½ teaspoon
- Cumin, ½ teaspoon
- Pressed garlic
- Lemon juice, ½ lemon
- Tahini, ¼ cup
- Sunflower seeds, ¼ cup
- Olive oil, ½ cup
- Cilantro, ½ cup
- Avocados, 3

What you will do:

1. Halve the avocados, take out the pits, and spoon out the flesh. Place everything in a blender and mix until completely smooth. Add water, lemon juice, or oil if you must loosen the mixture a bit.

> **4 grams – net carb**

> **41 grams – fat**

> **5 grams – protein**

> **6 servings**

Granola Bars

What you will need:

- Eggs, 2
- Sea salt
- Cinnamon, 2 teaspoons
- Vanilla, 1 teaspoon
- Tahini, 4 tablespoons
- Coconut oil, 6 tablespoons
- Dark chocolate, 2 ounces
- Shredded coconut, 2 ounces
- Flaxseed, 3 teaspoons
- Pumpkin seeds, 2 ounces
- Sesame seeds, 2 ounces
- Walnuts, 3 ounces
- Almonds, 3 ounces

What you will do:

1. Set your oven to 350. Combine all the ingredients in a food processor until coarsely chopped. Place this in a baking dish lined with parchment paper.
2. Let this bake for 15 to 20 minutes, or until golden. Allow it to cool a bit before removing. Cut into 20 pieces. Keep refrigerated.

> **3 grams – net carb**

> **18 grams – fat**

> **5 grams – protein**

> **20 servings**

Chocolate Hazelnut Spread

What you will need:

- Vanilla extract, 1 teaspoon
- Cocoa powder, 2 tablespoons
- Unsalted butter, 1 ounce
- Coconut oil, ¼ cup
- Hazelnuts, 5 ounces

What you will do:

1. Dry roast the hazelnuts until they turn golden. Make sure they don't burn. Let them cool slightly.
2. Rub the nuts in a kitchen towel until some of the shells come off. Those that don't are fine to stay on. Add everything, along with the nuts, to your blender and mix until smooth.

> **2 grams – net carb**

> **28 grams – fat**

> **4 grams – protein**

> **6 servings**

Zucchini Chips

What you will need:

- Taco seasoning, 1 tablespoon
- Coconut oil, 1½ cups
- Salt
- Large zucchini

What you will do:

1. Use a mandolin to slice the zucchini into chip rounds. Place them in a colander in your sink and add a lot of salt. Allow this to sit for 5 minutes, then press out the water.
2. Heat the oil to 350. Working in batches, drop the zucchini chips in a fry until golden brown. Set on a paper towel and sprinkle with taco seasoning.

> **2 grams – net carb**

> **14 grams – fat**

> **1 gram – protein**

> **4 servings**

Lemon Ice Cream

What you will need:

- Heavy whipping cream, 1.¾ c
- Erythritol, ⅓ cup
- Eggs, 3
- Juice and zest of 1 lemon

What you will do:

1. Separate the eggs. Beat the whites until stiff. Mix the sweetener and egg yolks in another bowl until fluffy. Mix in the lemon juice and zest, then carefully fold the whites into the yolks.
2. Whip the cream until it forms soft peaks. Fold the eggs into the cream. Add this to an ice cream maker and allow it to freeze following the instructions on your device.

> **3 grams – net carb**

> **27 grams – fat**

> **5 grams – protein**

> **6 servings**

Chocolate and Peanut Squares

What you will need:

- Salted peanuts, ¼ cup
- Cinnamon, 1 teaspoon
- Vanilla, ½ teaspoon
- Peanut butter, ¼ cup
- Pinch salt
- Coconut oil, 4 tablespoons
- Dark chocolate, 3½ ounces

What you will do:

1. Melt the coconut oil and chocolate in the microwave. Stir in the other ingredients, except the peanuts. Pour this into a greased casserole dish.
2. Allow this to cook and cover the top with the peanuts. Refrigerate. Once set, cut into squares. Store in the freezer or refrigerator.

> **4 grams – net carb**

> **12 grams – fat**

> **3 grams – protein**

> **12 servings**

Spinach Dip

What you will need:

- Lemon juice, 2 teaspoons
- Sour cream, 4 tablespoons
- Mayonnaise, 1 cup
- Pepper, ¼ teaspoon
- Salt, ½ teaspoon
- Onion powder, 1 teaspoon
- Dried dill, 1 tablespoon
- Dried parsley, 2 tablespoons
- Frozen spinach, 2 ounces
- Olive oil, 2 tablespoons

What you will do:

1. Thaw the spinach and squeeze out the excess liquid. Place in a bowl and stir in all the other ingredients. Allow the flavors to mix for 10 minutes before serving.

> **2 grams – net carb**

> **34 grams – fat**

> **1 gram – protein**

> **6 servings**

Baked Brie Cheese

What you will need:

- Pepper
- Salt
- Olive oil, 1 tablespoon
- Rosemary, 1 tablespoon
- Garlic clove
- Pecans, 2 ounces
- Brie cheese, 9 ounces

What you will do:

1. Set your oven to 400. Lay the cheese on a parchment-lined baking sheet.
2. Mince the herbs and garlic, and chop the nuts. Combine them with the olive oil. Add pepper and salt. Pour this over the cheese and let it bake for 10 minutes.

> **1 gram – net carb**

> **31 grams – fat**

> **14 grams – protein**

> **4 servings**

Salami and Cheese Chips

What you will need:

- Paprika, 1 teaspoon
- Grated parmesan, 4 ounces
- Salami, 20 slices

What you will do:

1. Set your oven to 450, or broil. Lay the salami slices on a parchment-lined baking sheet. Place cheese on top of each slice and sprinkle with paprika.
2. Bake until the cheese is bubbly and golden. Make sure they don't burn. Allow them to cool. Once cooled, they will be crunchy like chips.

> **1 gram – net carb**

> **15 grams – fat**

> **15 grams – protein**

> **4 servings**

Chocolate Fudge

What you will need:

- Dark chocolate, 3 ounces
- Butter, 3 ounces
- Vanilla, 1 teaspoon
- Heavy whipping cream, 2 cups

What you will do:

1. Boil the vanilla and cream together. Boil for a minute, then reduce to a simmer. Simmer until it reduces by half. This will take around 20 minutes. Stir occasionally.
2. Lower the heat again and add the butter. Mix until smooth. Remove this from the heat. Chop up the chocolate and add to the warm mixture. Stir until the chocolate has completely melted.
3. Pour this into a 7-by-7 baking dish and refrigerate until set. Sprinkle with cocoa powder and cut into pieces.
4. Keep this in the freezer.

> **2 grams – net carb**

> **12 grams – fat**

> **1 gram – protein**

> **24 servings**

Berries and Cream

What you will need:

- Vanilla, ¼ teaspoon
- Heavy whipping cream, 2/3 c
- Fresh berries, 1 cup

What you will do:

1. Beat the heavy cream until it forms soft peaks. Once almost there, add the vanilla. Serve the berries with a dollop of whipped cream.

> **6 grams – net carb**

> **29 grams – fat**

> **3 grams – protein**

> **2 servings**

Vanilla Pound Cake

What you will need:

- Eggs, 4
- Cream cheese, 2 ounces
- Sour cream, 1 cup
- Vanilla, 1 teaspoon
- Baking powder, 2 teaspoons
- Erythritol, 1 cup
- Butter, ½ cup
- Almond flour, 2 cups

What you will do:

1. Set your oven to 350. Add a generous amount of butter to a 9-inch Bundt pan and place to the side.
2. Mix the baking and almond flour, and set to the side. Slice the butter into small squares and place them in a bowl. Add the cream cheese. Place the cream cheese and butter in the microwave and let them heat for 30 seconds. Keep an eye on everything so the cream cheese doesn't burn. Once done, stir until the ingredients come together and are well-combined.
3. To the cream cheese and butter mixture, stir in the sour cream, vanilla, and erythritol. Make sure everything is well-mixed.
4. Pour this mixture into the bowl with the almond flour and mix well. Mix in the eggs one at a time, making sure each egg is completely mixed in.
5. Pour the batter into the buttered Bundt pan and place it in the oven, allowing it to bake for 50 minutes or until a toothpick comes out clean. If your cake still looks too wet, place it back in the oven for 5-minute intervals until it has cooked through. When touched gently, it should bounce back, but still have a bit of a jiggle. This is normal for desserts made with almond flour until they have cooled completely.
6. For the best results, allow the cake to cool completely for at least 2

hours, though overnight is better. If you take the cake out of the Bundt pan too soon, it could crumble a bit.

7. Keep this in the freezer.

> **5 grams – net carb**

> **20 grams – fat**

> **7 grams – protein**

> **12 servings**

Lemon Strawberry Cheesecake

What you will need:

- Strawberries, 2
- Zest of 1 lemon
- Lemon extract, 2 teaspoons
- Swerve sweetener, ⅓ cup
- Heavy whipping cream, ¾ cup
- Softened cream cheese, 3 ounces

What you will do:

1. Place the whipping cream, sweetener, and cream cheese in a bowl and beat together until they become creamy and smooth. Mix in the lemon extract, enough to evenly distribute. You can also add a bit of the lemon zest if you want a stronger lemon flavor.
2. Cut a strawberry into small pieces. Slice a second strawberry into thin, heart-shaped slices.
3. Fill 2 jars halfway with the cream cheese mixture. Add the chopped-up strawberry to the top of each jar to make a pretty layer. Add the rest of the cream cheese mixture to the top of each of these and smooth out the top. Top both with the strawberry slices, formed into a flower shape.
4. Sprinkle the remaining lemon zest onto the center of each of these strawberry flowers. You don't have to use all of it, just what you want.
5. Refrigerate these until you are ready to eat them.
6. Keep in the freezer.

> **5.3 grams – net carb**

> **48 grams – fat**

> **4.5 grams – protein**

> **2 servings**

Carrot Cake with Frosting

What you will need:

Cake:

- Melted butter, 1 tablespoon
- Ground cloves, ¼ teaspoon
- Ginger, ¼ teaspoon
- Cinnamon, 1 teaspoon
- Pinch salt
- Grated carrot, half
- Vanilla, ½ teaspoon
- Beaten egg
- Erythritol, 1 tablespoon
- Baking powder, ½ teaspoon
- Psyllium husk, 1 tablespoon
- Almond flour, 2 tablespoons

Frosting:

- Vanilla, ½ teaspoon
- Erythritol, ½ tablespoon
- Whipping cream, 1 tablespoon
- Cream cheese, ¼ cup

What you will do:

1. This is a mug cake, so grab a mug and mix all the cake ingredients in it. Mix everything together really well. (Ingredients like to hide in the edges of the cup.) If you want, mix everything in a separate bowl or with a blender to make sure it is well-combined. It also helps to spray the mug with cooking spray, so the cake doesn't stick.
2. Microwave the cake for 90 seconds. Turn the mug upside down on a plate to let the cake slide out and cool off. Once cool, slice the cake in

half and lay it to the side to cool.

3. Place the vanilla, erythritol, and cream cheese in a bowl and use an electric mixer to whip up all the ingredients so they form a soft and creamy frosting. Add the whipping cream and whip again for 5 minutes. Set this to the side.

4. Place 1 layer of your cake and scoop a heaping tablespoon of your frosting on it. Gently lay the other layer on top and scoop another tablespoon of the frosting on top of it. Use a spoon to spread the rest of the frosting over the cake any way you like.

5. Serve the cake now or let it chill before you serve it. The colder your cake becomes, the firmer your cream cheese frosting will be.

> **5.2 grams – net carb**

> **17.3 grams – fat**

> **5.9 grams – protein**

> **2 servings**

Blondies

What you will need:

- Walnuts, 2 tablespoons
- Chopped dark chocolate, ½ ounce
- Coconut flour, 2½ tablespoons
- Almond flour, ¼ cup
- Coconut cream, 2 tablespoons
- Vanilla bean seeds, 1 teaspoon
- Vanilla, 1 teaspoon
- Pinch stevia
- Erythritol, ¼ cup
- Dash salt
- Cream of tartar, ½ teaspoon
- Eggs, 2
- Coconut oil, 2 tablespoons
- Cacao butter, 6 tablespoons

What you will do:

1. Set your oven to 400. Place parchment paper into an 8-inch square baking dish. Measure all your ingredients.
2. Place the coconut oil and cacao butter in a microwave-safe bowl. Place them in the microwave for a minute and a half to let them melt. Take them out and stir them until no more lumps remain. If you must, microwave them for a minute more. Place this to the side to cool.
3. Using a hand mixer, combine the vanilla, cream of tartar, vanilla bean seeds, erythritol, salt, and eggs. Mix this for a couple of minutes, then pour in the coconut cream. Beat a few seconds longer until mixed well.
4. Add the cooled butter mixture into the egg mixture and beat until the mixture becomes dense. Depending on how cool or hot the ingredients are, the density could vary a bit and be anywhere from almost liquid to a creamy texture.
5. Place the 2 flours through a sieve and mix them together. Add these

flours to your cream mixture and fold it with a rubber spatula. Add the chocolate and mix together. If you want the nuts, you can mix them in now. Combine everything using a rubber spatula.

6. Pour this mixture into your prepared baking dish and spread the mixture evenly using your spatula. Place this into the oven and allow it to cook for 15 minutes. Once the toothpick comes out clean but they are still a bit juicy in the middle, the blondies are done. Don't over bake them.

7. Once they are cooked, take the blondies out of the pan and allow them to cool. Once cooled, slice them into 20 squares. These taste best the second day. They can be left in a container on the counter; they don't have to be refrigerated.

> **.7 gram – net carb**

> **7 grams – fat**

> **2 grams – protein**

> **20 servings**

Conclusion

THANK YOU FOR READING to the end of *Ketogenic Bible: The Complete Ketogenic Diet for Beginners*. I hope it was informative and that it provided you with all the tools you need to achieve your goals, whatever they may be.

The next step is to grab your shopping list and head to the grocery store. Once you have everything you need, start the 14-day plan. Within those two weeks, you will learn more about your body and how the keto diet affects you. You will probably drop a few pounds in the process as well.

Finally, if you found this book useful in any way, a review on your favorite book retailer is always appreciated!

.

Made in United States
North Haven, CT
18 June 2024

53790990R00098